HOUSE CALLS

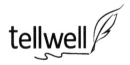

Tellwell Talent

www.tellwell.ca

ISBN

978-1-77370-412-8 (Paperback)

HOUSE CALLS

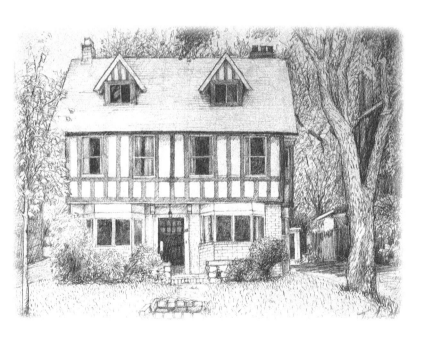

DAVID SMITH, MD

INTRODUCTION TO HOUSE CALLS

This is a collection of short 'vignettes' recalled from my earlier experiences while studying and practicing medicine in the late forties to the mid eighties.

It seems now the home visit is making a comeback. Practitioners have rediscovered the benefit of the encounters in the patient's home environment. Primarily so in the care of older patients, but also in pediatrics and general health care. So much can be learned by observing the living conditions, which in many instances may have major implications in managing their care. Primarily safety factors re elders – clutter, lighting, the deadly 'scatter rug', smoking, health and fire risk. A look in the medicine cabinet or side table may indicate outdated or over-the-counter medications or old prescriptions which need to be discarded! Also, one often finds unnecessary 'supplements' or other highly promoted remedies (usually useless), wasting money better spent on good nutrition.

The patient's financial status, a major factor in determination of health, might be better observed. The patient may arrive in the office dressed in 'designer clothes', but living arrangements suggest otherwise. This information would not be so easily documented in a routine office encounter. The doctor-patient interaction is certainly enhanced and strengthened.

In the past few years, the outreach of 'palliative care teams' with the newer perhaps more acceptable term 'supportive care', can keep the patient out of hospital, surrounded by family and friends in their home, closely supervised by community care services to effectively manage fragile and end-of-life care.

Thus, the house call may prove to be of some benefit in improving the general health of our communities, urban, suburban and rural. How does society manage a large complex, bureaucratic, politicized organization? My conclusion after many years of practice… start by improving home care!

David R. F. Smith MD., CCFP., FCFP.

TABLE OF CONTENTS

INTRODUCTION TO HOUSE CALLS 4

WHAT IS LOVE?. 7

THE POWER OF PRAYER 12

THE GUN 17

HAPPENINGS 20

MEDICAL ETHICS 28

THE DUCHESS 32

CONNECTIVITY. 37

A HOTEL CALL 41

THE HOSE. 45

COMPLIANCE 51

THE LEGEND. 57

NO WAY OUT. 62

MEMORIES OF THE DEPRESSION 75

DECISIONS 79

BAD MEMORIES 85

SHOW BIZ 92

SEX-ED FOR THE COMMUNITY 99

A REALLY BAD CASE OF MEASLES 106

NORMAL MORE COMMON THAN ABNORMAL. 112

A TALE OF TWO POLICEMEN 118

UNIVERSITY ADDRESS. 123

EPILOGUE. 127

ACKOWLEDGEMENTS 129

WHAT IS LOVE?

I was seated at the small kitchen table with a faded oilcloth cover, I had just filled out the death certificate and called the funeral director. It was a Saturday morning, so I was concerned there might be a delay. Elizabeth, the deceased's wife, sat quietly staring out the window. I had an awkward feeling of sadness, so to fill the silence, and with nothing immediate to attend to, I told her I would wait until the funeral home attendants arrived. "Would you like a cup of tea?" she asked. "Thank you," says I (I hate tea), so the gas hissed and the big kettle went on the stove.

Wei Fei (Wally) Leung had died of lung cancer. As a lifelong smoker, he suffered from chronic obstructive pulmonary disease. I had treated him for pneumonia several times in the past, and was concerned about his deteriorating condition. It was impossible to convince him to have an X-ray as it would mean a trip to the hospital which he would have to pay for. This was in the early 1960s: no insurance and the concern re costs of illness loomed large. Also, health maintenance was not considered in those days as the doctor was only called when the patient was truly ill. Thus, when hospital admission was rejected, patients elected to stay at home. As Wally gradually deteriorated he was never neglected nor did he ever complain. They seemed appreciative of what care I could give, and the devotion of this couple was quite amazing.

As an inexperienced new family physician, I was getting an early introduction to palliative care. Her care, as I noted, was outstanding. They had no children, relatives or even close friends. The apartment was immaculate: the bedding was always clean and neat; there was fresh water, a clean towel and a basin for expectoration by the bed at all times. She carried on, week-in and week-out, for several months, alone!

As I was remarking on this, she looked at me as she poured the tea and said, "You know, doctor, I never really loved my husband." I was stunned! How could a person demonstrate such care and devotion without love? She, aware of my confusion, started her story…

Elizabeth, born in England, obtained a position with the British Military Command in Shanghai, China in 1935, as a stenographer, bookkeeper and assistant manager. Wally, a Chinese national, was closely involved with the military base arranging for supplies, as he was a local importer. He was a pleasant man and well-liked, and was in constant contact with the military base staff. At the time, Elizabeth was romantically involved with a young British officer stationed in the compound. Now, this is the point when the Japanese had begun aggressive expansion by invading China, and by spring of 1937 the danger was imminent. Indeed, by June 3, 1937, the actual invasion of the city of Shanghai was taking place. Elizabeth was distraught, having lost all contact with the active garrison as the military had been dispersed as active defenders. The Japanese navy was shelling the city and it was chaos. Wally showed up at the compound and urged her to leave at once. She was reluctant to leave without any contact with her beloved officer, but it quickly became obvious: leave or perish! My memory shot back to my childhood. In 1937, I had just turned eight years old. At that time kids were able to buy penny candy and gum. With the gum came cards, some featured hockey or sports figures, but some depicted the horrors of the war in China: gruesome bomb explosions, bodies thrown in the air, atrocities! As a kid, these cards left an indelible memory; horrors that haunted me. I could only imagine the terrible distress those involved suffered.

Wally finally convinced her to leave and he was able to find accommodation on a freighter bound for Vancouver,

Canada. They escaped the bombardment and blockade and made their way safely across the Pacific Ocean. Now, those were the pre-war years of the Great Depression and few job opportunities. As they had very little money, Wally, through connections, got some work, but they were also in a difficult situation trying to find an acceptable place to live. As a mixed-race couple who were not married they were constantly rejected. Thus, they agreed on a marriage of convenience. Finally, Wally got a job in Toronto, so they moved and settled there and have lived quietly all these years in a drab third-floor walkup apartment on upper Jarvis Street.

I stared down at the teacup, fine bone china, showing its age by the tiny tea-stained mosaic of cracks; tea leaves scattered at the bottom. Wally had died with dignity in his own home, as he wished. Elizabeth continued to stare wistfully out the window. "He was a kind, caring, devoted man and I know he loved me. No one could ask for a more compatible partner. But oh, to go back to those wonderful days before the war." The funeral home staff finally arrived. I felt a lump in my throat and tried not to let them hear the catch in my voice. I suggested that I should inform the woman next door with whom she was acquainted that Wally had died. She indeed came right in to see Elizabeth and seemed very supportive.

I returned home and gulped down a mug of coffee to eliminate the taste of the tea. I looked at my wife and my baby son who had waited patiently while I was on my house call, and we finished breakfast together. What is love? I've never forgotten that couple.

THE POWER OF PRAYER

In 1980, I had started working on the sixth floor of The Salvation Army Chronic Care Hospital in central Toronto at one of the new palliative care services that was then being developed. These were collaborative groups introducing the "Circle of Care", that is, physicians, nurses, physiotherapists, occupational therapists, dietitians and chaplains of various denominations. The concept of total care was evolving; medically, socially and spiritually. This was a learning curve for me as I had always considered end-of-life care to be not well managed, and this was a great step forward.

One of my patients, a woman in her late sixties, was in end-stage cancer of the colon. Her pain had been well controlled, but as she was slowly deteriorating her main problem now was extreme fatigue. She was lucid, however, but she seemed focused on a loose-leafed binder, the type used as notebooks in school. I had become only slightly aware of this and had paid little attention to it. One day, she presented it to me, asking my opinion about its possible usefulness. I was uncertain what to say, but did encourage her to complete it if she could. Over the next few weeks she worked assiduously to complete a documentation of her illness.

On my second-last visit to her, she proudly presented me with this truly surprising account. I had been previously rather dismissive, but when I realized the meticulous care she had taken in producing this journal, I was impressed. I was also taken aback at the accurate documentation, which she had started shortly after the onset of her illness, and her perception of the medical reports and information from a layman's point of view.

I must say, I did try to read some of this at her bedside, realizing this was not something just to be perfunctorily set aside. I took the journal with me and later, at the nurse's station, I sat and started to read. I had to take it home to completely absorb it. This was truly the story of a medical failure. Years later, screening for colon cancer would be heavily promoted. In her account, there was no assignation of blame to herself or the medical profession, it was simply a chronicle of what happened. She wondered, if her anemia had been noted earlier, would this have helped? She was unaware of any relatives with this disease, but she had come from central Europe after the war as a young woman, with no knowledge of her family history. It was immediately obvious she had put enormous effort into this endeavor over the past months. It suddenly dawned on me that this lovely, always-pleasant woman, whose complaints were minimal for a person so ill, was managing her illness with a positive approach: no self-pity, no remorse, just an effort to make a difference. Not for herself, but hopefully for others.

Now I was faced with a dilemma. This was a compilation of information that was of immense importance to her. Of what importance would it be to the medical profession, and how was I to give her some assurance that this was truly of help to others? Well, it turned out it was of use to me! As I continued in active practice, I intensified my search for colon malignancies. That is: following up re anemia, using rigid scopes (as there were no flexible scopes at that time), and taking bowel X-rays. As a result, over the course of my career I was fortunate in discovering successfully-treatable colon cancer in a significant number of my patients, including parents of two of my best friends.

On my last visit, she eagerly asked my opinion about what should be done with her journal. I told her I had read it all (I had, although it took some time), and that it would certainly affect my practice patterns, and hopefully that of other physicians, as I was in a faculty of medicine teaching facility. I indicated that I would request medical records to include this information. Being the time it was, they reluctantly acquiesced.

As we completed this discussion she suddenly grasped my hand with her pale, thin, cool fingers. "I am so relieved and grateful that you encouraged me to finish this, I was afraid you thought I was wasting your time." "It's OK," I murmured awkwardly, because at that time I had no idea of what would become of the journal. Then, tightening her grip, she earnestly requested: "Pray for me?" Holy Cow! Where was the chaplain when I needed him? Now, I did have a religious upbringing as a kid; church on Sundays, Sunday School (my aunt was the Sunday School teacher), but I had drifted away from religious ways over the years. How to manage this? I was OK with the Lord's Prayer, but after that? I tried to think of all the recitations from church, funerals, even weddings that I'd heard over the years. I somehow got going after starting with the Lord's Prayer, carrying on for several minutes, recalling nothing of what I had said. But I did try to say it as reverently as possible.

Unbeknown to me, the nurse attending the patient in the other bed (behind a curtain), heard the request. She had evidently gathered the available staff who had then located themselves outside the door. They heard it all! The patient released her grasp and closed her eyes, weakly thanking me. She really seemed at peace. Well, as I left the room I was greeted with gales of laughter. I was immediately nicknamed "Reverend" and teased, a few of them suggesting I was in the wrong profession.

The following day I received a call from the head nurse. She reported that the patient had spent a quiet night, but had deteriorated during the morning and had died at noon in no apparent distress. Lesson learned. My determination to aggressively pursue the diagnosis of colon malignancy was stimulated. The fact that I had read the journal and told her it would be a matter of record (albeit buried in an old, archived medical record system), somehow legitimized her efforts which had, I believe, a very profound effect on the last days of her disease. Whether or not the prayer helped? Who is to say? Certainly not me.

THE GUN

I strongly dislike guns! In my mind, it's because of the incredible harm they have brought to mankind. Disclosure: at age 14 I did possess a single-shot bolt-action rifle for the purpose of shooting groundhogs, crows and rabbits. I am not proud of this activity, although very little harm resulted from my adventures: six groundhogs, one rabbit, no crows.

In the sixties, I was the physician on call at the Royal York Hotel. It was early in my career and I was fairly inexperienced. In those days, there were no 911 calls; the doctor was summoned and expected to attend to the problem. It seemed there was a hotel guest who was causing a disturbance by crying and calling out constantly. The night manager had been called and determined that this gentleman was likely in need of some sedation. Hence, the call for a physician. When I arrived, the door of the room was partly open; the night clerk, the security guard and a housekeeper were awaiting my solution. I quietly entered the room–which was only partially lit–to see this man pacing back and forth, alternately crying and cursing in a rather incoherent way. It took me about five seconds to notice that he was carrying a gun! I, as noted, was only slightly familiar with long guns, so assessing the type and nature of what appeared to be an automatic pistol was daunting. In that moment (when I should have run out and called the police) I reverted to the words of my psychiatrist teacher: "ask and listen."

"Is that a loaded gun?" I questioned. "Ya…ya," says he. "What do you intend to do with it?" "Kill myself!" he replied. "When will that be?" "Soon, soon," he replied, in a completely dispirited manner. I quietly spoke: "Why on earth would you want to do this?" He sat down on the edge of the bed and I sat opposite him on the other twin bed. Through sobs he started to describe what led up to this crisis, all the time waving the gun around. I was getting disturbed that he might accidentally fire the gun, so I said: "Please give me the gun before you shoot me or yourself!" To my amazement, he gently handed me the gun. As I had never handled a handgun I was surprised at how heavy it was. I thanked him quietly and said: "I'll get rid of this now if you don't mind," and he acquiesced without resistance.

I immediately ran out to the hall and handed the gun to the security guard, who I thought would be comfortable with firearms. Not so! He dropped the gun as if it were a hot potato; luckily it did not go off! I returned to the room and sat down opposite him again. For the next three-quarters of an hour he recounted a heart-rending story of addiction, failed business and a totally destroyed family, ending in what he considered to be "the only way out." Sobbing, he said: "I've even failed at that." As a businessman in the US he was a victim of poor judgement, ineptitude and bullying by associates, along with family dysfunction. He recognized that his plan to come to Canada to end his life was another wrong step in his most unfortunate life. After a period of tearful, almost childlike reflection, he agreed to be sent to the psychiatric service of the hospital at which I arranged admission. He, to my relief, accepted my suggestion. As the ambulance attendants carefully gathered his belongings he–emotionally and physically exhausted–collapsed on the stretcher. As he departed, he grasped my hand and said: "Thank you for listening, no one ever listened to me."

HAPPENINGS

She was smart, funny and feisty, and one of the best women athletes at the University. She was my friend. We had met at the Toronto Lawn Tennis Club. She was an outstanding young player, I was a middling player, and we were paired together in a club doubles tournament. Thanks to her we won the first few rounds, but thanks to me we were finally eliminated. She was very tolerant of my efforts and aware that I was beginning to reduce my playing time due to the fact that my early medical practice was picking up momentum. She enjoyed ribbing me about anything medical, and had a supply of doctor jokes handy at all times! She did not seem to be overly impressed with the health care system, in that her only recent contacts were with orthopedic surgeons. She had experienced several sports injuries and had a hard time complying with their rather patronizing admonitions re "safety in sports", especially with respect to women. I don't ever remember winning when we played squash (she was the club women's champion) or tennis, and although I often felt she was toying with me, I did at times come quite close. One sport I could do better than she was swimming, as she tended to sink (due to high body density), and she appreciated the fact that I had swum competitively, giving me some status as a so called athlete. The large tennis / squash group at the club enjoyed several years of great fun, lots of gamesmanship, kidding and good competition.

One of my medical responsibilities was working at the University of Toronto Student Health Service. At this point in time, I was fairly junior in the service and was bothered by the system, in that the sexes were separated; women upstairs, men downstairs. The program at that time was run on the military model, as most of the senior physicians were recently retired from the Canadian Army Medical Corps.

One afternoon, I heard a raising of voices at the front desk. I then heard a rather loud female voice stating: "I want to see Smith." Not accepting the fact that all women were to be sent up to the women's division, the male receptionist, although very confrontational, could not convince her to comply. As my door was open, I scurried out to the desk. There was Trudy, my tennis buddy. I defused the situation.

"Come in," I said, to the great irritation of our receptionist, who saw service in the invasion of Italy as a first-aid man, and was a stickler for rules. Following me to my office, she said: "I gotta see you, I have a problem." Closing the door, I asked: "What is it?" She leaned forward earnestly to speak, and I had that "Oh-oh" feeling one gets in this profession. Never one to mince words: "I have a lump in my left tit!" She had found this while showering a day ago. "What do you want me to do?" I asked. "Jesus, I came to ask you to tell me what to do," she replied immediately. She was always free with profanity.

Dilemma: as I was not her regular doctor, I asked who was. It turned out that the last doctor she had seen other than through sports medicine was her pediatrician, who had dismissed her at age eighteen! I gently suggested she have one of our female physicians see her and advise her on the best plan of management. She would have none of that: "I'm asking *you*!" When offered, she refused to see a nurse from upstairs, so I asked her to get on the examining table, and when she complied I threw a sheet over her. On examination, there was revealed to be a significant mass medially located in the left breast. I was surprised she had not noted this before. Also, I detected a small lymph node on the left axilla (arm pit)! It did not help matters when she recalled that her grandmother had a "breast problem", which was never discussed by the family. I tried to be casual in stating that this will need further investigation. Fortunately, in those days my call to the surgeon was answered immediately, and as he came on the phone I tried not to sound alarming, but I had to impress upon my consultant friend that this was rather urgent. He read me loud and clear. As it was almost 5:00 p.m. he said: "I will see her tomorrow at 2:00 p.m. I'll fit her in." I reassured her that this was the best plan, and I explained this would require a surgical biopsy, and that the surgeon was very competent in this field. Well, the expected followed, this was a very malignant tumor with a very bad prognosis. Surgery, radiation, follow up; but she did not really come to the realization for some time that the prognosis was bad and her chances of survival were practically nil. In those days cancer was a disorder not easily discussed. As I visited her in hospital and followed her post-operatively, as well as in the ensuing weeks, I realized she wanted to know about her prognosis, but had so far not asked. This woman was just in her twenties! She was a fighter; she wanted to do absolutely everything to attack this disease.

I had very little experience with a malignancy with such a poor prognosis in so young a person, made worse by the fact that she was only slightly younger than me (she was actually the same age as my wife, another keen tennis player and also her friend). I had always been troubled by the avoidance of open discussion between patient and doctor when facing such a diagnosis. No mention of approaches to counseling management re bad news really appeared in our curriculum. How to handle this? The surgeon, a very conservative yet compassionate man, had not broached the subject of bad prognosis, as she had not asked. "The tumor and lymph nodes have been removed and we will have to wait and see." Radiotherapy was to ensue.

After she had finished her therapy, I took the opportunity to sit quietly with her and talk. She had already indicated that I was to be her doctor. Her parents and her brother seemed to concur, and proved to be incredibly supportive throughout her illness. I started by asking her what she thought her response to treatment was, so far. She was coming to the realization that progress was not as she had hoped. Knowing her appreciation for straight talk, I told her my opinion: this was almost certainly to have a fatal outcome. "Oh, SHIT" (her words). This short and unpleasant expletive, so often used in everyday mishaps, eloquently expressed the fears, hopes and anxieties, as well as the horrible realization, of the situation she faced. Silence, then with a long sigh she thanked me for being honest and forthright, admitting she was arriving at the same conclusion. She was discharged home. I admitted

I did not know how long it would take, but I assured her that I would not ever abandon her.

She progressed slowly through the early fall but finally developed pleuritic (chest) pain, and then bone pain, both due to the spread of her cancer. On a day that I was not on call the pain became severe, and the family took her to the emergency department. She was admitted under the surgical service, where she was assessed by the surgeon and his resident. They agreed with my suggestion that this was a bad prognosis, stating that there was nothing more they could do. Morphine was prescribed. This was to be administered every four hours around the clock in specific amounts. This was standard procedure. On her third day in hospital the pain was worse. After lunch, I went to the floor to visit, and see how she was managing. The complete surgical team had just arrived: the chief surgeon, a 'visiting fireman,' (vernacular for other than hospital medical staff) the resident staff, interns and nurses. I stood at the door as there was no more room at the bedside. "How is she doing?" the surgeon asked the head nurse. "Don't ask her, ask me, 'cause I'm not doing OK! Jesus, Doc, you've got to give me more morphine!" The response did not surprise me. "You must be careful with such powerful medication, I would like you to hold the present dose as we don't want to cause harm, we will monitor your response." "Is that it?" says Trudy. "Yes," he replied. She shot back: "Then you can take your morphine and stick it up your ass! I won't take any more if it's that bad." Silence. In those days, such a response was unheard of. Nervous coughs, shuffling of feet, then the entire retinue left the room. "We will discuss this further," was muttered as the group left. In the hall, my friend the surgeon quietly said to me "I would be pleased if you took over her care from now on."

I went back into the room. "Way to go," I said, almost punching her arm (it was actually a poke on the arm, a favorite custom of hers). We talked, she apologized for mouthing off. "Don't apologize one bit," I said. I felt sorry, in a way, for the surgical team who were just following established protocol in limiting the administration of narcotics; this was something that really troubled me in a situation such as this. I arranged with the head nurse, with whom I had a good relationship, to change to another narcotic to maintain the no-more-morphine request until her pain was fully controlled. Pain control was fairly adequately maintained, but, unfortunately, she did not get to go home, as further complications arose. But she had time with her family and close friends before she died quietly seven days later on Halloween.

Two days before Christmas, a parcel arrived at my door. "Sign here," said the man delivering what appeared to be a case of wine. My wife appeared beside me, curious. I opened the envelope inside. It simply said: "Thanks for getting me through this… Trudy." We both choked up. It took quite a while to drink that wine, every sip bringing memories of great times. Later, I discovered her brother had arranged this at her request!

Not too soon afterwards I got a chance to attend a conference on a topic not previously presented to the U of T Medical Faculty. Dr. Balfour Mount, a physician at the Royal Victoria Hospital in Montreal, was proposing a new approach to palliative care (a topic not often discussed), i.e., the management of end-of-life care, initially in cancer patients, but later to encompass any terminal disease. This program promoted maximum achievable symptom control, an all-embracing concept of total care which included not only the patient but family and friends; taking into consideration medical, social, financial and spiritual concerns. Everything one needs to depart this world with dignity. With Trudy in mind I signed up, starting a lifelong interest in this field. I am glad to say that many years later this discipline is strongly promoted in Primary Health Care.

MEDICAL ETHICS

I had only been practicing for a short time when I received a call from one of my teachers who was aware that I had established an office in downtown Toronto. I was rather impressed, as he was requesting I attend his housekeeper. I was surprised that he would consider me for this endeavor as I had not, in my opinion, been an outstanding student, managing an average middle-of-the-class standing. He was a highly respected lecturer, a senior clinician at the teaching hospital and a fount of knowledge on a wide range of medical topics. We had all experienced his quiet but intense quizzes which even the best students found intimidating.

This man was a bachelor, who lived alone in a large Victorian house on a quiet street downtown. This home was impressive, in that off the entrance was a room–obviously a library-cum-study–lined with books and a table literally loaded with medical journals and scientific publications. Intimidating! His housekeeper, I was informed, was from Northern Ontario and had been in his employ for many years. She had a sister and a cousin as her only relatives. Her quarters were on the third floor: a small suite, sparsely furnished.

She was sitting in her chair by the bed, she was pale and thin, and looked exhausted. Her present complaint was indigestion, loss of appetite, abdominal pain and marked fatigue. She expressed concern, as she felt she was not properly managing her duties. After an examination which included a simple hemoglobin test (which was slightly low), not much of significance was detected. She was, in a general sense, not well. After some discussion about her work and her state of mind, it became apparent that she was quite depressed, having heard that her sister, whom she had not seen for almost three years, was also not well. Her work entailed care of this rather large house, and although there was a cleaning lady who did laundry and a man who did all the manual labor, she was responsible for meals and administration. The doctor was away a lot and spent a great deal of time at the hospital, so hers was a very lonely existence. Her gastric problem would have been considered in those days to have been possibly due to peptic ulcer disease. Tea and biscuits or baking soda partially relieved the symptoms. However, it was the concern and stress and also her age (early sixties, although she did appear to look older) that impressed me. I enquired when she had last had a vacation to visit her relatives. It was actually three years since she had been home last. She had Sundays and partial days off mid-week, and her social life was comprised of church functions, but she had no really close friends.

It seemed apparent to me that she needed some time away from this rather dismal and demanding work, so I asked her if she had considered a vacation in the form of a trip home. Her reply was that she felt that she was really needed here, although she admitted she would very much like to "get home for a while." I asked if I might suggest she take some time off, perhaps go home, which I felt would be truly helpful. It had become obvious that she was very devoted to her employer, being so reluctant to abandon him. I persisted, however, and was given permission to request that she have some time off. In the meantime, a simple diet was suggested and a different antacid preparation was advised. I returned to the study, where the doctor awaited me, and sat on the edge of a large leather chair. Now I faced my former teacher with trepidation. I must keep in mind that the nature of the illness and her medical condition were not for me to divulge; confidentiality was paramount. He was the employer! How to proceed?

He opened the conversation with generalities: "How did you find her? I have been concerned for some time.

It would appear she has a gastric problem." I could sense he was about to launch into a discussion concerning her medical status, perhaps one as he was accustomed to; a bedside conference. However, after a moment's hesitation, he thankfully refrained, and then asked my opinion. I also sensed that he had a genuine concern for her welfare. Speaking generally, I noted she was very tired, and had expressed concerns about her performance. I also felt he should know that there were no true signs of significant concern which would require hospital admission. An X-ray and further blood tests would be helpful, and I would arrange this. But I also suggested–and she had given permission for this only reluctantly–that she have some time to travel home and spend some time with her family. To my great relief he immediately concurred, stating that he had become oblivious to the fact she had always been available, constantly adjusting to his irregular schedule and his often fastidious needs.

As the tests were not indicative of significant disorder, arrangements were made, interestingly by his other significant employee, his hospital secretary. Train tickets and travel, as well as four weeks of time away. As I finished my encounter, he said, almost to himself: "Why didn't I think of arranging some time off?" Wow! Imagine that coming from this outstanding man. At that point, very early in my career, I felt that I had arrived.

THE DUCHESS

I was totally unprepared for what I was about to experience on this next house call. Ascending the steps of the impressive Victorian mansion that had recently been converted to a rather luxurious nursing home, I was wondering how my encounter with the Duchess would turn out. These visits were always interesting. I had given my relatively-new patient this moniker as she was a product of the Roaring Twenties, that was her time as she had been born in the late 1800s. Now in her late 60s, she would never reveal her true age. The head nurse at the facility had asked me, a new family doctor in the community, to take over her care.

Her history was interesting. She was married in the thirties to a man of some wealth, social status and military heritage. He was an officer in the Canadian army who, when war broke out, was assigned overseas. He was unfortunately killed in action toward the end of the hostilities. They had no children, and she was left with a considerable inheritance. During the periods prior to and during the early part of World War II, they lived an extremely active social life in the upper echelons of Toronto society: parties, balls, Royal Winter Fair, horse racing, etc. Having smoked heavily all her adult life, she had, over a long period of time, developed chronic obstructive lung disease, and had recently been in hospital where it was discovered she now had widespread carcinoma of the lung.

I had some trouble getting the hospital records. She had been admitted with pneumonia, and it was noted that she had had several episodes in the past. Biopsy of airways revealed malignant cells. She was told she had a serious lung condition, but the word "cancer" had not been used! Her previous MD, quite senior to her and at the point of retirement, had told her she would have to leave her rather large and luxurious apartment as, although she had a maid and houseman, she would require more intensive care; hence the move.

On my second visit, having obtained the necessary information, I brought up the diagnosis, and, of course, used the word "cancer". She was upset that the older doctor had treated her as a child! Now our plan was to follow a palliative trajectory which depended on the progress of the disease. She was glad to hear that we would not plan another hospital admission unless absolutely necessary. I discussed possible oxygen use, as it might help with her difficult breathing, but when she realized she would have to give up smoking it was clear that this was not going to happen. She was, of course, allowed her evening intake of Scotch whisky (Johnny Walker Black Label).

Our relationship slowly improved, she of course thought of me as a child (at age 28!), but she finally accepted me, and as a result I was rewarded with anecdotes from the twenties and the war years, gossip re the Toronto Establishment and opinions on politics with which I was not always in concordance.

Now she was gradually worsening: further weight loss, some increasing pain and respiratory distress, as expected. Over the past several months it had become evident that she was failing fast. The most recent insult was incontinence requiring a diaper.

It was always an experience entering her room. First, one was assaulted with the smell of cigarettes, she had defiantly continued to smoke although she could only take the occasional puff before an exacerbation of distressful coughing. She had always used a cigarette holder about five inches long, held between thumb and index finger, palm up. She somehow thought this would protect her from the harmful effects of smoking! The room also reeked of strong perfume, the expensive kind. Her industrial-strength make-up was now not so meticulously applied, a change for her. Now, imagine a composite of Gloria Swanson, The Duchess of Windsor and Greta Garbo: faded elegance, well past her prime, but wonderfully defiant! Her demeanor had earned her the nickname Duchess, which by now I and the nurses had adopted, and she seemed to accept this, perhaps in deference to our admiration of her spunky attitude toward this dreadful disease.

I had just completed my examination: not good findings. I was about to start a discussion re further plans of management, she adjusted her silk pillow with some difficulty, looked at me intensely and said, "Hand me that leather folder on the dresser." With careful deliberation, she opened the folder and produced a checkbook, and said to me: "I will write you a check for ten thousand dollars… If you will kill me. Now. My life has become intolerable! Every shred of dignity is gone. I am going to die, we both know that. I am relegated to wearing these goddamned diapers!" With that she pushed down the covers, revealing her emaciated body swaddled in a damp diaper. "I will NOT put up with this nonsense any longer! DO YOU UNDERSTAND!!"

Wow! I sat stunned, but in reality, I did understand. My sister's dog had to be put down recently for an illness less ominous than hers. Until recent times the consideration of euthanasia was that it was totally unacceptable and illegal. But after barely one year in practice this was more than my annual income! I took her hand and said: "Put down the pen. We both know I cannot do this," although I did admit it was a reasonable and tempting offer. "You'd end up dead, and I'd end up in jail. OK for you, not good for me!" She sighed, "Oh well, I won't apologize for trying." I reassured her we would really work to control her symptoms, and reminded her that she wore diapers when she came into this world. Gallows humor, which she accepted with grace.

Over the next short period she did deteriorate, then slipped into a coma and died quietly. Her only relative, a niece living in Montreal with whom I had only spoken to on the phone, came to Toronto to settle her affairs. She told me, as I had suspected, my patient, The Duchess, had been a legend in her time.

CONNECTIVITY

I had been in general practice for barely one year, discovering daily what I had not learned in medical school.
A call had come from a woman pharmacist I had known
mostly through contact by phone. She had been helpful
with counseling several of my older patients with respect
to managing complex dosage protocols while taking
multiple medications. It was back then that I began to
appreciate the role of pharmacists in such a process. We
had met once in the store while I delivered a narcotic
prescription; she was a fairly young professional who had
just recently graduated, and she impressed me with her
knowledge, as well as her interest in her clients. She stated
she was reluctant to bother me, but had a request: could
I visit her mother, who had just learned she had become
fairly ill. Glad to comply, I arranged to make a house call
that evening.

It was January-cold and snowing. With some difficulty I found the house: an older home, a rooming house in the Annex. A small light on the porch barely illuminated the number. Cranking the bell (before electric doorbells), I finally heard the door start to open. I was met on the porch by a small, slightly stooped, grey-haired man, appearing tense, wearing only light clothing and a thin sweater. I asked if we could step inside, but he stopped me and insisted he pay my fee before I saw the patient! I implored him to step in from the cold, and it *was* cold. In the vestibule, he opened his purse-like wallet and extracted seven dollars, as I had told him at his request that was the fee for an evening house visit. It almost seemed that he could not trust me to treat his wife without prior payment, this was confusing to me.

We climbed to the second floor where he and his wife had a small suite, furnished in the European manner with lots of lace and tassels; they were obviously immigrants who had come to Canada after the war. In his strong German accent he introduced me to his wife, Sophie. Sitting propped up in bed she looked obviously ill even in the darkened room, and she appeared to be very tense and apprehensive. Her husband had moved to the side of the bed, standing as close as possible with one hand on her shoulder in an extremely protective way. Usually in those days it was the accepted practice to examine the patient without the family member(s) hovering. It was apparent this was not going to happen. Body language indicated he was barely able to allow me to conduct a proper physical examination. After completing my history and physical examination it was obvious she had pneumococcal pneumonia.

Upon informing them of my opinion, i.e., that she had pneumonia, they seemed to clutch each other almost in panic. I tried to explain that treatment would very likely be effective and it took a great deal of reassurance to even partly calm them down. I was able to administer an initial injection of penicillin and assured them that I would arrange to have their daughter organize the prescribed oral dose, assuring them I would follow her response to this medication. He repeatedly asked: "Will she recover?" as he sat holding her, his arm around her shoulder. As best I could, I reassured him. At that point, I realized that I should inform the daughter and they were very glad to have me do this.

I was able to contact my friend the pharmacist, first to let her know what I felt to be the problem, and then to order the oral meds through her pharmacy. Upon remarking on the fact that they seemed so anxious and concerned, she stunned me with their story. There had been no indication from my history-taking that there had been previous problems, indeed she had stated that she had never been ill, and was evasive about discussing past health problems. It turned out that she and her husband were the only members of both of their families to have survived the Holocaust, having been liberated at the war's end. They had, with great effort, made it to Canada and had their one daughter ("for us a miracle"). Subsequently, they admitted having had many health scares, both infections and injuries during the terrible ordeal that they somehow endured, thus the diagnosis of pneumonia was to them a possible death sentence.

This was my first encounter with any survivor of the Holocaust. As a child and teenager, I had only experienced the war and subsequent years by following the news and recounted stories. Of course, we were horrified and enraged by all of it, but it took the experience of dealing with two human beings who were so bonded and connected by their past to even begin to comprehend the enormity of the societal effect of this human tragedy.

A HOTEL CALL

"Nuts." Another night call from the hotel. The night clerk had informed me a woman had been found unconscious about midnight, and asked if I could come and see her. I slipped quietly out of bed so as not to disturb my wife and put on my clothes; at that time suit and tie was the correct attire. Button-down shirts were helpful, tie already on shirt, (faster), suit on rack, etc. I often wondered if a fireman's pole would be of help.

In those days, no 911, the doctor on call would respond. I arrived and was escorted to the room by the night clerk. Actually, the room was a full suite, very luxurious, fit for Prime Ministers and the like. In the reception area, scattered over the chairs and sofas, were open shopping boxes and parcels, luxurious articles of expensive clothing and shoes, some littering the floor... It looked like Christmas! I was led to the bedroom, and across this huge bed was the inert body of a woman. It was immediately apparent she was alive and breathing. She had presented lying face-down, and with the help of the clerk and a housemaid I was able to reposition her so once she was examined all vital signs were intact. It appeared that she was drunk, or possibly drugged, as she did smell of alcohol, but not heavily so. No evidence of trauma was apparent, i.e., no blood or marks of injury. When I tried to arouse her with a painful stimulus she partly came to, and with a string of the foulest epithets told me where I should go! She could be aroused, but then just fell back into a deep sleep. She was unable to give any verbal information.

Now, this was no ordinary individual. First, her hair was died bright red, but not like a normal redhead, it was fire-engine red and there was lots of it! She was extremely attractive, one would have assumed Hugh Heffner would have chosen her as his chief Bunny. Wow! At that instant, a man appeared from the bathroom carrying a handful of pill bottles. He was a huge guy who could have been a character in The Sopranos: rumpled silk suit, Gucci shoes; he smelled of alcohol and seemed quite annoyed and not really concerned about her present state. It seems they had had a quarrel and her anger had not been placated by the shopping spree. He led me to the bathroom, which was a mess: spilled cosmetics, powder, perfume, eye make-up… But most notable was a message in red lipstick on the mirror: "Fuck you… you will find me dead." I felt I had staggered into a Mickey Spillane story. It took some time to rifle through her train case and effects to try to ascertain what drugs she might have taken and when.

As it turned out she had thankfully taken no barbiturates, all were forms of benzodiazepines, mostly Valium. I recorded this, estimating a toxic, but not likely lethal, dose. The night clerk had contacted the ambulance service. I supported the order as it would be inappropriate to let her stay in the hotel to recover. As the ambulance arrived, she again partially awakened to express her opinion of first her male friend, and then the rest of us present, in her usual blasphemous manner, then off she went. Before I left the hotel, I discovered that this lady was a famous former stripper from Chicago. Her moniker was "Flame Fury" and her friend was her manager who saw to it that she met the right people. In other words, she was a very high-priced hooker who generated a substantial income. She was evidently well known to some prominent people, no names, of course. I had called the ER at my hospital to make them aware that an overdose was arriving, the triage nurse was not happy but had no choice. I said that a note would accompany her re my findings and any drug information. I did not get to speak to the doctor who was on call. Finally home, I quietly slipped off my clothes, put on my pajamas and crept silently into bed. I wondered what the guys in the ER would think of this remarkable lady.

Suddenly my wife awoke and rolled over. She sat up in bed, exclaiming: "My God, where have you been?" Although I had thoroughly washed my hands and face I was unaware of the fact that I still reeked of cosmetics and perfume. In order to make an impression I told her I had an interesting encounter and that it was not cheap perfume. The humor escaped her, so she went back to sleep.

I, however, was wide awake; I was bothered by the fact that, in spite of her apparently affluent and exciting life style, she was obviously miserable enough to attempt suicide. Her manager had told me after she had left that this was not the first time she had tried this, she always did it when she could not get her way!

When I later enquired how my patient was received in the ER that evening, none of the staff were too pleased, as she was not a cooperative patient and certainly not amenable to counseling with respect to lifestyle, healthy sexual practices or any other behavioral modifications. So after a miserable night in the ER she finally woke up and stormed out, not demonstrating one morsel of appreciation for the care provided. I imagine being a courtesan with all its attendant risks perhaps outweighs performing on stage, where she got her start. The two women residents who were responsible for her care in the ER were not amused.

THE HOSE

They seemed the perfect couple. She was cute, attractive in a very wholesome way. She was a figure skater, good enough to compete in free skating, figures and dance. Her best performance was in the dance competition. I was somewhat surprised he did not even skate, but was evidently a good golfer, and was quite successful as a young executive in a new business venture, his forte being accounting. I became involved through a friend from the skating club who had long been an acquaintance of mine; he suggested me as a new family doctor. She seemed pleased to learn that my younger sister and I had competed–albeit at a lower level than she–in figure skating dance competition. I had seen her on several occasions re minor conditions: colds, flu and a minor knee injury. I had never met her husband, I assumed he was not in need of my medical attention and was very busy. It subsequently turned out he had a family doctor who also attended his parents.

It was almost one year into their marriage when tragedy struck. I had not seen her for some time when she presented at my office complaining of a gradually-increasing lower back pain, rather non-specific. She looked well, as usual, and so far this had not affected her skating. I, of course, assumed this was as a result of her rather active life-style. Examination did not suggest a sign of musculoskeletal injury. But there was a minimal finding of some slight local swelling in the mid-back, right side which I could not explain. I prescribed aspirin as there were no good nonsteroidal anti-inflammatories in those days, and asked her to cut back on the intensity of skating practice.

She was to return for follow-up in two weeks, or sooner if it worsened. She returned, but at this visit she was no better, and the discomfort was possibly a little worse. Now she noted she thought she felt "something in her mid-back on the right" Reviewing my notes, the area where I had thought there was a thickening, on really careful examination, revealed a soft ill-defined mass, not red or warm to suggest infection, but associated with some discomfort on pressure. What was this? Now, this young woman was tough and not a complainer, rather, she was playing down her symptoms. I had a seat-of-my-pants feeling that although I had no idea what the underlying cause was, I had better pay closer attention.

She was referred to a general surgeon, a very competent man, who, following his first visit, stated he was also baffled by the findings. I was glad to hear that he had noted this unusual finding, and to my relief suggested we pursue this further, and that he would arrange hospital admission. The long, sad story unfolded slowly as there were no CTs or MRIs in those days, and it took some time to finally discover that she had a very malignant kidney tumor which had spread posteriorly through the muscle layer and had positioned itself in such a manner that surgery was unlikely to be in any way effective in achieving a cure. Biopsy confirmed the diagnosis.

This set off a sequence of painfully bizarre events. I was upset to notice that when she was in hospital her husband visited only for very brief periods; this was strange. It turned out that he had a severe phobia re hospitals and illness; he could barely get himself into the area of her hospital room, and left after the briefest of visits. This, of course, caused her great distress, and she became angry and upset, not able to understand his behavior. He was totally unable to discuss her disease, seeming even more distressed than was she! We tried to explain to her that his inability to cope was an emotional response, but it was to no avail. Her family was extremely supportive, but also became extremely intolerant of his behavior; I knew this well as I had dealt extensively with them following the diagnosis. I had no direct contact with his family, only with him in an effort to help him cope, but as I was not his doctor I was limited in the ways I could make a difference. The patient and her family were coping as well as could be expected, they were fortunately sustained by a strong religious faith, and came to accept the prospective outcome. She had tremendous support from her skating community, from the church and from many friends from work and surrounding neiborghhood.

Now came the conflict! She suddenly stated that the marriage was over. Strangely, he was less responsive emotionally. The next phase was to split the assets. They conjointly owned the house, and started the painful disposition of house and contents. Oddly, he now seemed to be more responsive, not to her, but to the whole situation. He appeared relieved to be out of what apparently to him was an intolerable situation, one which was beyond his capacity to emotionally handle. But, accountant that he was, he started counting! Now, although she was quite ill and was undergoing palliative treatment, she was determined to carry on the negotiations.

When I had occasion to be in the neighborhood I would drop in to follow her illness. I pulled up in the driveway to discover the house had been sold, and I was rather horrified to arrive at a time when this divorcing couple were arguing over the contents of the garage! All the garden tools were out and spread around: lawn mower, shovels, etc., and a very long garden hose, required for the extensive area of gardens surrounding this attractive home. He seemed to want the hose, noting that as she was now living with her parents she did not need it. I could hardly believe this was happening, considering the circumstances. "Hi Doc,"she called out to me, "I'll be with you in a minute." Then, with resolve, she picked up a pair of garden clippers and, pulling the hose out from its reel, laid it on the driveway and cut it in half! I stood stunned by my car, its door still open. She came over, got into the passenger seat, sat down and started to cry. We sat in the car with the doors open on this hot summer day; nothing was said for several minutes. She dried her tears and apologized for losing it, we looked over the mess in the driveway: tools spread all over, a little trickle of water from the severed hose darkening the pavement. "He was just so damned precise, I could never reach him, and when I needed someone, he just cut and ran!"

I felt there was no use trying to explain that he was cursed with obsessive and

phobic problems, which would require intensive therapy to manage. She had enough to deal with on her own. We talked quietly about skating, we looked at the hose and started to laugh and laugh, tension released.

Her parent's car pulled up and she thanked me for the visit (during which there was no discussion about her illness). I drove off wondering if she actually took her half of the hose.

COMPLIANCE

She was what my grandfather would have called an ample woman. As the matriarch of an extended Italian family, she was an imposing figure. Mrs. A was a mother, grandmother and great-grandmother. Her dominance over the large family was impressive. The problem was her unwillingness to adhere to any suggestions that would ameliorate her deteriorating health. She was the typical complex-care model that primary care physicians are so often called upon to manage. She was obese, although not morbidly so, she had Type II diabetes, was hypertensive, and suffered progressively arthritic knees and hips. She and her deceased husband, who had come to Canada as young adults, had followed in the family business of pasta-making. The business had been sold due to the fact she could no longer manage as CEO and none of the many younger members were willing to take over.

This left a rather overbearing, imperious, now-retired woman; still very mentally alert but resentful of her reduced mobility re stairs, who was now free to devote her time to the full administration of the family. This had resulted in my being requested to take on her care as she had dismissed her previous physician, an older doctor who had attended her family, including her husband. The family felt he was a good doctor, but Mrs. A expressed to them the fact that he had not saved her husband, who had died suddenly of a cardiac death. Though not much could have been done in those early days with no organized awareness of what we now consider cardiac risk factors, as he was a heavy smoker, ate heavily, drank a lot of his homemade wine, was averse to any form of exercise, and, I am told, was exposed to a lot of stress.

As I was already caring for several members of the younger generation, they decided that perhaps I could attempt to manage Grandma. As a young physician, I was willing to accept a new patient. I was, of course, concerned re my ability to get her to go along with my care plan, as I was just slightly older than her granddaughter! Of course, it was obvious that she, and her late husband, were not amenable to medical advice. I subsequently heard through the hospital grapevine that her former physician was somewhat relieved at this arrangement.

At my first encounter with my new patient, having been introduced by several family members (all well known to me), I became aware of her intense scrutiny. Looking at me, assessing my age, dress and new medical bag (of which I was rather proud), she addressed me as her family members gathered around the bed: "So you my new dottore, you not so old? My girls say you OK." She sat upright in her large ornamental bed, bolstered by many pillows, wearing lovely ornate European style bed clothes. Wow! The word "imperial" seemed to fit. However, beyond all this there lurked a twinkle in her eye and a subtle tone of humor. I wondered if I could somehow win her confidence and thus some modicum of cooperation.

"May we get started?" I asked, requesting that the daughters leave us alone. "They try to push me around," she stated. I figured it would take a bulldozer to push her anywhere! First the complex history: medical, family, sociological; extensive. Then the physical examination. Next, I perused the array of pharmaceuticals displayed on the side table, some only partly used, some empty; a big challenge. Finally, after finishing my assessment (and with some difficulty), I reduced her meds to the minimum and eliminated the sedatives. At least she was happy to stop the sedatives: "They make my head funny." I left her. "May I tell the girls about the changes and plans?" Which, of course, included dietary advice. "Sure, you tell, but I might not listen."

Our relationship grew, through lots of give and take. Here, the art of achieving compliance was so apparent. Not: "What are you going to do for me?" rather: "What are you going to do for yourself?" Needless to say, her willingness to follow my advice was rather poor. Her love for food was her downfall, try as I might to get her to reduce the intake, and while she swore: "I no eat nothing!" no apparent weight loss ensued.

I had to finally admit defeat. On one occasion, I was called to see her as she had "suffered a spell," according to her daughter. This came mid-morning, on what was not a good day for me. The night before I had been up most of the night with a very slow first baby, which finally delivered (fortunately free of complications); home to bed at 5:00 AM; slept in; missed breakfast; coffee only; just made it to the office. My nurse fielded the call stating that, as the spell had passed, I would not have to leave at once but would come at noon hour (lunch), as soon as my morning office was done. I arrived not much later to find no signs of any neurological deficit or stroke, but I was concerned about this occurrence which was not well described or observed. The patient was demonstrating no signs of distress, and was also alert, so the pressure was off. Keep in mind, at that time no ultrasound or other more advanced investigative procedures were available. She, sitting in her chair, watched me closely as I conducted the examination. "You no look so good, you tired." I muttered: "I didn't get much sleep last night, I had to deliver a baby." This (a mistake) brought on a flurry of sympathetic outbursts from what was now two daughters as well as the patient. "You no eat-a?" True, I had not had, nor had I much thought about, breakfast, and lunch was looking improbable at this point. Mrs. A took over! She sent a daughter downstairs with a torrent of instructions in Italian, the other daughter also departed hastily. She reached forward, and pinched my cheek, then gave it a gentle slap. I was sitting on a stool beside her chair, caught off guard. Seeing my mild embarrassment, she said: "Dottore, you fix me, I fix you!" Footsteps on the stairs; suddenly there appears before me a tray with a huge dish of steaming spaghetti with meatballs! Well, it did look good! I must say, to be polite I tasted this, cautiously. It was delicious; what could I do but eat? Boy, my family often made spaghetti, but never like this. While enjoying this wonderful food I suddenly noticed the granddaughter had appeared and placed a large glass of red wine on the side table. Oh-oh, now what? I had to get back to the office and finish a busy day! I simply could not refuse, so I just gave in and finished this superb food. Reluctant as I was to drink the wine (I was not a wine drinker), I must admit this was the smoothest glass of red wine I had ever encountered. I had cleaned the plate, wiped my chin on the white linen serviette and commented on the excellence of the pasta, when to my complete surprise another plate of spaghetti arrived from the kitchen below. I did eat some more, but soon reached my limit. As nicely as I could I thanked the girls and congratulated Mrs. A on the family's culinary skills. The estimated calorie intake must have been well over 2000! What if my family was having spaghetti for dinner tonight?

The afternoon passed, albeit with me in a somewhat soporific state. My receptionist asked: "Did you have a chance to get lunch?" My reply: "I grabbed a snack," then disappeared back to my office, checking for spaghetti stains on my tie. How does one lecture a family on dietary restraint when such delicious fare is available? My gulping down a plate and a half of this great food, plus wine, kind of disqualified me from pontificating on eating habits. Good food is a blessing and a curse! Over the past years medical science has struggled with the problems of food and nutrition, and will continue to do so for years to come. How to feed over seven billion people, not too much and not too little, with minimal waste? It's as big a problem as climate change!

Mrs. A lived for several more years, finally suffering a massive stroke, gone in a very short period, no suffering. For years afterwards the various family members and I remembered with great humor this remarkable matriarch, whom I dubbed "The Queen of Dundas Street West."

THE LEGEND

This is a mildly embarrassing vignette. It really depicts the rather old-fashioned attitude toward sexuality in the early fifties. In fact, during our four medical undergraduate years, no teaching at all was provided with respect to sexuality or any form of contraception. Our rather resourceful class group had arranged talks on birth control and its various methods provided by none other than the companies who produced condoms and diaphragms and other very unreliable products. These presentations were of only questionable help, in retrospect they were actually often misleading. Our older classmates were mostly married men who had been in military service who, apart from raunchy jokes, were not very forthcoming with useful information on sexuality.

My partner and I were on our first rotation on the urology service in our first year of internship. Both being unmarried and not having steady girlfriends we were lacking in worldliness, truly clueless by the standards of today. However, we, as did most of our younger contemporaries, had hope.

The previous night I had admitted a man in his mid-sixties. He was in total urinary retention, in considerable distress and requiring catheterization, which, with the help of the senior resident, I was finally able to achieve. He was a large, fit man, of apparent Scandinavian descent. He had a very enlarged prostate gland, and admitted he had a progressive history of restricted ability to urinate. He was admitted, catheter in place, and after the next two days after work-up it was determined that he should have a prostatic resection. In those days, before the advent of universal health care, he had been admitted to the public ward and was charged the minimal daily tariff for the bed, while his medical care was provided free by the residents and interns, and supervised by the appointed teaching staff. Also during that period, the wait times were minimal, as the demand on the health care system was somewhat restricted by the fact that there were much fewer procedures for both investigation and active treatment, and people were expected to pay for medical services unless unable to do so.

The chief resident was anxious to get on with this plan, which would enhance his surgical experience, so surgery was set for the next day. The patient was given the explanation for the urgent need to open the urethral tract, and was warned of the possible consequences of the procedure. He was made aware that a careful check for malignant disease would be conducted and that there "could be some interference with your sexual function in the future." At this point he became agitated, deviating from his previously stolid, imperturbable demeanor. He pleaded that this operation be delayed or even postponed. However, both the resident and the attending surgeon impressed upon him the necessity to proceed. He reluctantly complied.

His post-operative course was uneventful, with catheter in place he was instructed that in due time, when the bleeding was controlled, the catheter would be removed and he would be discharged. He later called me back and seemed very interested in the workings of the catheter, and I naively explained that the rubber bulb at the tip was inflated, thus preventing the rubber tubing from slipping out, and that there was a clip on the tube leading to the bulb to keep it inflated.

Another two days passed, we stopped by regularly to see that he was progressing as expected. The catheter had just stopped passing significant amounts of blood, I had said: "Good sign, when all clear, you will be out of here," and went off to complete rounds. Now, he had been encouraged to get out of bed and walk the length of the ward: twenty-eight beds surrounded by curtains with the nurse's station centrally located. He could even walk in the corridor if he felt able. Upon my return, I noted he and the small trolley to which the catheter and urine collection bag was attached had left for a walk. One hour later I returned, the curtain was closed. I paid no attention. As I was leaving the ward for the cafeteria, the curtain was still closed.

During dinner, I was called to pick up an urgent message. When I called the number given I was surprised to hear a very agitated woman's voice with a strong Scandinavian accent: "He iss home! He iss home, vat can I do, he is bleeding quite a lot!" It took me a minute to realize that this was my patient's wife. Somehow, he had left the hospital unbeknownst to the nursing staff and had taken a taxi home. Fortunately, they lived only a very short distance from the hospital. "Bring him back immediately," I ordered, "Get in a cab and come at once."

They arrived in the ER and he was immediately transferred back upstairs. It appeared he was able, with my description of how the catheter was designed, to deflate the bulb, pull out the catheter and, as he saw only a small amount of blood, figured he could go! Well, we reintroduced the catheter and admonished him for his behavior. His distraught wife asked quietly if she could speak with me alone. In the private room, she told me the following story. They had been married for fifteen years, she was his second wife, the first wife had left him. He was a hard-working man, a house-builder, recently out of work. She then recounted her problem. Since they had been married, he had insisted they have sex on a "regular daily basis!" At first, she said: "It was OK, he use condoms back when I have period. But every day, he very healthy man, hardly ever sick. Now I don't want, he never hurt me, but cries and begs so I give in. Now he home, he tries to have sex, says he must have! Too long time to have no sex for him." Of course, this prompted the recurrent bleeding.

Well, in my wildest dreams, I could never imagine such a situation. I told my partner this story at lunch. He said, "Wow there's hope for us yet!" The chief resident just said: "I don't believe it." The poor patient did not notice the large number of male residents and interns who just casually wandered by to have a look at 'The Legend.' The nursing staff treated him with some distain. This was the only case of prostate surgery where I felt that if he did have the side effect of sexual dysfunction it would be no great loss! Just think, his poor wife had just had five days off!

NO WAY OUT

"There's no way out, I will have to kill myself!" I was truly stunned by this outburst. This was a dilemma which, for me, was unprecedented. How was I to manage this complex, long, heartbreaking story, which had no possibility of satisfactory outcome?

My patient had been an easygoing man of roughly my own age. He had a good job as an executive, with kids and an attractive professional wife. They lived in a nice area in an interesting house. They seemed to have it all. I did not see him often, as I was more likely to meet him on the subway than in the office. However, he appeared one day, having recently made an appointment for no stated cause. But as soon as I saw him I could tell he was not the man I had known for several years. None of his usual upbeat demeanor, no sign of his usual daily joke; all humor just gone. He did not look well. He had had his annual physical just over one year ago, and at that time all was well. His past history was very unremarkable: bad flu once, occasional bad colds, sprained wrist (squash): a healthy, fit, active man. To complicate this presentation, he was vague and seemed unable to describe his presenting symptoms. This in a usually bright and decisive senior executive. He had stopped squash and quit bridge club, stating he was too tired and, besides, he had lost interest in many of his usual activities. He had also lost some weight, as he was less interested in food (he was evidently a good cook). This, of course, suggested a depressive episode, however, he denied episodes of depression either in himself or his family. He could not at this point come up with any explanation for his present state.

I immediately arranged for his return for a complete examination. Blood work was ordered, including thyroid and lipid screen (his father had history of heart disease), as well as a chest X-ray, as I noted he had a very slight but persistent cough. He had only traveled on business in Canada and the US, never in northern territories or tropics. Anticipating problems in figuring out this problem, I had booked extra time. However, after a very careful examination and review of the blood work and chest X-ray, no abnormal findings were apparent. He had lost five pounds (he was lean to begin with), but had a strange, almost gaunt look which was made more remarkable by his flat affect. Could all this be associated with an endogenous depression? Was this true pallor? He was not anemic. Continued questioning did detect some problems with his business, but he seemed reluctant to discuss this. My "ask and listen" approach did not seem to get a response. He seemed to be uninterested in a more intense follow-up, but I insisted. Further blood work was ordered. I had quietly enquired about sexually transmitted disease, his response was: "I guess you could try that."

So, the work-up continued. However, all the investigations provided no answers. To make matters worse, he did not improve, but continued to lose weight, and neither did his depression improve. He declined anti-depressants, but finally decided to follow my suggestion that he be referred to an internist, who, after seeing him, like myself admitted he did not yet have an answer, but would admit him to hospital–as was the procedure at that time–to further investigate. As my practice was appended to the hospital I was easily able to follow his progress daily, as an inpatient. After three days and much further investigation, no specific diagnosis was made, but it was apparent he was not in any way improving.

Now, it happened that at that time a new medical resident had just come on service. This young doctor was an American who had just left New York City where he had been a resident at Belleview Hospital. We were talking in the hall and he asked if he could follow up on a hunch. During his experience in New York he had become aware of an unusual new disorder noted in gay men in the downtown area in which they developed a progressive disease associated with wasting, loss of weight and markedly diminished resistance to infections, as well as unusual lung disorders and rare skin malignancies. This disease had a bad prognosis. He also noted that our patient seemed to demonstrate this pattern! He asked if this man was gay; I told him I didn't think so, but anything was possible. He asked if we could send a blood sample to the CDC Ottawa lab to be tested for this immune deficiency disorder.

At this point he was discharged back to my care pending the outcome of this test. My responsibility was to pursue his sexual history and any possible exposure to this disease. The internist (infectious disease) felt that as I had known this man and seemed to have his trust, I should follow this. The results finally came after a two-week wait. I had only told him that a very special test was being conducted and that this investigative procedure was totally new to me, so I would have to await the results, and that the medical team would follow up when the information was available.

We spent the next two weeks awaiting this report. Now, this was the early eighties, HIV testing was only done in one lab in Canada. The US Centre for Disease Control did not start the routine testing for this virus until mid-1985. There was little doubt that this major government lab was reliable. In fact, they routinely retested all specimens to ensure accuracy. Unfortunately, this test did not become routinely available in Canada until November 1985. My patient arrived at the office after the results came back. I had booked one hour, and I was having a very difficult time facing this encounter.

He was told that he tested positive for an unusual disease and that it was transmitted by sexual contact or by unsterile needle use. And that the usual sexually transmitted diseases had been tested for, and no evidence of them was detected, I asked if he had any idea how in the world he had contracted this disease. Stunned silence, then, head in hands, he recounted this heartbreaking story. "Jesus, how could I have let this happen?"

As a young engineering student, he had enjoyed the usual beer drinking, partying and high-jinks so character-istic of the times. He fell in with a group of older students who to him were impressive, as they were very socially active; an elite campus group, very involved in sports and extra-curricular activities, most were very outstanding students. He wanted to be part of the group. One guy in particular whom he admired–very handsome and artic-ulate–was a winner of several student awards, some for outstanding academic achievement. He hung out with this gang through second and third year; what a time! He had been brought up in a very strict family so this was liberation for him. Early on he had made some unsuccessful attempts at seducing girls and one event had completely discouraged him. Awkward advances, poor situation (i.e., roommate could arrive home any minute), prospective partner very apprehensive, no proper birth control in place: disaster! She cried and he was totally embarrassed, he just could not do it! Back to the frat house where the guys were hanging out, where he foolishly confessed to his lack of success. This was followed by endless suggestions, they plied him with beer. He was now fairly drunk, totally dejected, and alone with one remaining person: the guy whom he had always admired. This man was amazingly sympathetic, pouring another beer and suggesting that maybe he was not really cut out for sex with girls. After all, some people can have sex with someone of the same sex, or be bisexual. He somehow produced some very pornographic exotic magazines and suggested they try some stuff. The rest of the evening was a blur; he recalled some sexual contact. He was embarrassed and confused but got home, and missed the next morning class, having the sense that what had happened–while somewhat sexually satisfying–was probably not good.

As examinations were approaching, this was the last of the partying and revelry. He was a good student and determined to do well, so all social activities were suspended until the exams were over. As he had a summer job out west and he was leaving immediately, he did not get to be involved in post-exam festivities. Upon his return the next year, all his former pals, being a year ahead of him, had departed, and he realized he had better get down to serious work, and as a result he graduated with honors. He finally did succeed with women very well, got married and had children.

During the ensuing years, he had a successful career, and had become a senior partner in his firm. He also had become aware that a large American company was poised to take over the company in which he was involved. As well, he knew that the president of this American firm was none other than his formerly admired "friend". The merger was undertaken; he was invited to New York to be involved with the reorganization of the new company. There were meetings and several social events. On one occasion, he was there without his wife as she had very important business of her own in Toronto. The night following the meetings, there was a party in the very impressive Manhattan Towers condo of "The Boss". As the party ended the guests left, and as he was about to go his friend asked him to sit down and have another drink, as he had a very important offer to make. Accepting another Scotch (he was no longer a big drinker), he listened to what was offered. It was proposed that he be installed as president of the new Canadian division of the firm. More Scotch was poured. Then, reminiscences followed by glowing memories of the great times they all had back at university, more Scotch, then the seduction really started. With the result: "I just rolled over, fell back on the huge couch… I was really out of it! How could I have let this happen?!" He got back to his hotel, and finally home.

Adjusting to his new position was distracting and extremely stressful , but he was finally partially able to put this encounter out of his mind, and to try to get on with his life. Over the next eight years, he had managed to do this. However the gradual onset of this inexorably progressive disease had finally become apparent.

Now the problem of prime importance was his home sex life. His wife, in her stressful job and juggling work, parenting and menopause, had in the past (fortunately) been intolerant of oral contraceptives due to severe migraine headaches, so birth control had always consisted of condoms. Also, as she had developed gynecological issues, during this period their sex life had "just evaporated". Following his New York experience, he had avoided any further personal contacts with his "friend", always arranging to have his wife accompany him when in New York. This awful encounter (for both of us) lasted well over the hour. He slowly sat back, and in a desperate tone pleaded with me to, under no circumstances, reveal this information to anyone, even his wife. This was of great concern to me as she would need to be tested. I reluctantly agreed: "for now". As I had been so absorbed in this story I had taken very few notes, and explained I would, of course, maintain total confidence. For now.

Now the threat of suicide. I explained to him that his plan to have a fatal fall or car accident would not answer the plan of confidentiality, as with any violent or possibly self-inflicted death the coroner would be involved and hospital records would be requested, thus, the diagnosis would be made available to the next of kin. I extracted an absolute promise that he would not consider this plan, and he assured me he understood the futility of going ahead with it. I arranged for close follow-up. Just imagine, only days ago I had been wishing for something other than colds, flu and crying babies!

The next day his wife called me, insisting I take the call at once; I did. She was upset and I was apprehensive about what her husband may have said. "You still don't have a diagnosis?" Well, no," I replied, evasively. "Therefore, I'm taking you off this case and will have him see another doctor, do you understand?" "Is he willing to go along with this?" I asked. "He will be," was her reply, and she hung up. His wife had her own physician, whom I knew, and she was the one who was to take over this case and "solve the problem". Several days later, she called. "What is going on?" she asked. I explained that while we had spent some time on this illness and obviously were dealing with a progressive disease, "J" had explicitly instructed me to maintain complete confidentiality, even to his family. I also explained that we were waiting for some further testing by an outside lab to complete the assessment. This was true, as there were confirmatory tests ordered (the Western Blot). "I'm sorry, that's all I can say now, good luck with your work up." Now, this woman was a first-rate family physician, bright and very up-to-date. As hoped, she picked up on my comments. I was sure he would not be likely to repeat his story to her as he knew her to be a friend of his wife's, and would still be very concerned about confidentiality. She sensed, upon my mention of awaiting a 'confirmative test' from the Centre for Disease Control in Ottawa, the provisional diagnosis. She did follow up with another assessment, as requested. She handled this delicate situation extremely well.

He came back, keeping this original visit with me, having not yet informed his wife. He still looked gaunt and ill, he remained depressed. How could he not be? I informed him that I would attend a conference on this new disease being held at UCLA Berkley, to gain as much information as I could. He was to go along with his new medical assessment and only provide information that he felt he was comfortable with. Now I started trying to persuade him to tell his wife and family what had happened, a major problem for me as I had a duty to inform his wife, who would require testing. Sooner or later they would find out the full truth, and it would be very much better if it came from him. Still, he could not bring himself to do this, but I told him I would keep in close touch and follow his progress in spite of his wife's objection. He was encouraged to work on nutrition and activity, which for him now meant daily walking; dietary supplements were introduced. I felt antidepressant medication would likely not make much difference. He was starting to have trouble at work, so it was finally decided that he take time off. As this would not affect his financial situation, he complied.

A few days later I received a telephone call at 3:00 a.m.! It was his wife. I snuck into the den to take the call and over the course of one hour of conversation (having first berated me for not having told her), she slowly began to understand that this was a case of sexual assault in a strange situation of power, charm and coercion, strengthened by an offer which was incredibly attractive! Finally, she began to understand. She had extensive experience as an executive dealing with Human Resources, and had become aware of the many instances of women in her employ who had suffered sexual exploitation and abuse who were unable to adequately resist and subsequently suffered the feeling that these occurrences were somehow their fault. She was aware that her husband was extremely interested in advancing in the business, but was not truly an aggressive person (a trait expected in CEOs), and that he tended to be more compliant in his administrative management style. This actually made him more appreciated by his peers, who had been distressed by his apparent deterioration.

Now came the "how could I have not traveled with him?" More guilt; she was choked with tears. Man, do I remember that absolutely gut-wrenching encounter! The problem of the incredibly busy, upwardly-mobile people is that they are constantly overwhelmed by professional, economic and family demands and can be vulnerable to a societal accident, usually an illness, injury, substance abuse or other misfortune. This was a very unusual and horrible medical disaster, one of the worst I have encountered in my many years of practice.

We followed his case to the end. It was established that the perpetrator of this problem had indeed left the company some years earlier for health reasons. I had returned from the HIV conference in California, having been assured that casual contact was not a risk of transfer with the virus, so when my patient had been admitted for the final time, succumbing to an overwhelming lung infection, I was able to visit him several times in hospital where the protocol was still gowns, mask and gloves.

Disdaining these, I was able to shake his hand and give him a hug. I sincerely told him how well he had managed to finally handle this unfortunate occurrence, and that fortunately his wife had tested negative. He died peacefully two days later.

A recent encounter with the former head of infectious disease at the hospital recalled those early days before the anti-retroviral drugs had become the standard to control (not yet cure) HIV, he claimed they were the most horrible years of his career!

MEMORIES OF THE DEPRESSION

One day, when I was in first pre-meds in 1948, I was reminded of an encounter I had in the fall of that year. On the campus, I met with a childhood friend, also entering U of T. We had played together as kids during the mid-thirties, his family was suffering the terrible effects of the times. His father, an engineer, had lost his job. His mother took in laundry, his sister baby-sat; but they had survived, and were now living in Leaside, a nice neighborhood. His sister had just graduated from U of T; they had made it through!

Memories flooded back to the mid-thirties when I was about seven years old. Times were tough, my father had just started medical practice in 1927, then the crash came and it became very hard for people who were ill to afford medical care. My father was often unable to collect bills owing, but we did manage comparatively well, as he would often be paid in products or services. I can recall the many men who came to our door begging for some help or food, offering services in return. I recall their appearance: partly shaven but always dressed in suits, shirts and ties–albeit very unpressed and disheveled–but, in their desperate way, attempting to maintain some dignity. Some wore woolen caps (we later called these "po-man's caps", as in the Roots hats for the winter Olympics), or the alternative, a battered fedora. My family tried to offer help, and my dad devised a simple solution. He would supply my mother and his nurse/secretary with a handful of signed prescriptions. If they were impressed with the supplicant's real needs, the individual would be given a script which could be taken to the local tea room, actually a small restaurant beside the local pharmacy. Here they would be provided with a hot meal, a slice of bread and a cup of coffee. Each Saturday morning, my dad and I would walk down to the corner where the pharmacy and the restaurant were located. My father would redeem the scripts, each worth thirty-five cents, paying the owner for ten or more, which pleased him and relieved my mother, or others in the house, of feeling like they had to try to provide food or money. The restaurateur, who was also a patient, would augment the offerings when he could. Some of these desperate men had a rather frightening appearance, and as a result we kept a baseball bat behind the door. Now, what could a small boy or a woman do in case of an attack? However, not once were we ever threatened or treated with disrespect. The gratitude of these men (as they were, in our experience, all men), was remarkable.

Years later, during the war, a very respectable man in army uniform appeared at the office door. He stated that he just wanted to come by and thank the person who had provided him with a meal when he was down. He was very pleased for the opportunity to meet my father, who at the time was in the Canadian Army Medical Corps and stationed in Canada. Dad invited him in for tea, they chatted, and this man told him that when he was in Winnipeg he met a man who told him that if you are ever in Toronto there is a place where you may get the benefit of a decent meal.

My father laughed, because on one occasion, while standing in the window watching the men go from door to door requesting help, he observed one individual who, after consulting a ragged piece of paper, walked directly to our house, checked the address and approached with his request for some assistance. This time, as my father was present, he answered the door and questioned the man as to why he came directly to our house. "Well, sir," he began. He said he had not stopped at the other houses because he met a man in Winnipeg who told him: "A kindly man at this address in Toronto might provide a meal." Our visitor laughed, as he had come to Toronto during the Depression in a vain attempt to get employment, and finally had to return home to Winnipeg. "You know, I suppose that was likely me." He told us that on the soup line, endless gossip about any form of help was the constant topic of conversation. How word gets around!

This encounter so impressed me as a high school student. My father, the aforementioned "kindly man," inspired me as I entered medical school. He emphasized that while you may not be able to cure a patient, you can always be kind, polite and respectful. I think that through the years many people have failed to comprehend the enormity of the Dirty Thirties and the effect it had on one's self-respect. Down-and-out was the situation of so many good people. Unfortunately, it was the horrors of world conflict that dragged the world out of the Great Depression.

DECISIONS

"Just get me a god-damned doctor!" I could hear this very insistent background voice on the phone, which my wife was holding. She had called me seeking advice, and was speaking quietly as there seemed to be a problem where she was working. The call had come from the Canadian National Exhibition stadium dressing room. There was a big-time entertainer in town and he was about to perform (this was for a single performance), the stadium was starting to fill up, and the warm-up musicians were preparing to go on shortly. The problem was that the star attraction had lost his voice! The producer of the show had exhausted all his contacts in attempting to have a physician come to assess the situation. Obviously, very few doctors would be keen to answer such a request as it was late in the day, approaching 7:00 p.m., and the willingness to accept responsibility (especially in a situation such as this) for a GP was unlikely. It was completely out of the question to get an ENT (ear, nose and throat) specialist on such short notice at this time of day. "Just go to the emergency department," would be the only response. My wife was a publicist at that time, assisting with the promotional planning, and someone in the organization knew she was married to a doctor. Hence, the quiet phone call from her while standing in an adjacent room: "Could you help?" Well, as it happened, I was attending the evening clinic at The University Student Health Service, which closed at 7:00 p.m. After she explained who it was and the nature of the problem I was very reluctant to offer to help. I was also aware that my good friend, an ENT doctor, would not likely comply.

My wife was sounding desperate: "All he needs is an injection. Is that so hard?" Well, to me that was a red flag! What kind of an injection? Who was to order this? The performer, well known to me and practically everyone else, seemed to be in a state. When I informed the nurses as we left the clinic that this guy wanted a shot, they both volunteered immediately!

I was finally, albeit reluctantly, coerced into going in order to, at the very least, assess the problem. The pressure was mounting as there had been episodes in the past when big-time performers failed to show, sometimes riots had erupted, with thrown chairs and screaming fans causing disruption. An example was the Alice Cooper cancellation in 1980.

With great trepidation I set off, my wife having stated it was the only option. I arrived at the administration parking lot as instructed, and was immediately whisked off to the stadium in a security car.

Upon entering, I could hear the loudspeaker announcing a temporary delay, with an accompanying roar from the crowd. As I entered the large dressing room area, confused activity prevailed. The producer, a big man of powerful demeanor, seemed to have little concern for the performer, famous as he was. He had been instructing the warm-up band to extend their stage time, he then directed me to the star's dressing room.

Now, here was the situation. This man had a rather bad head and chest cold. Runny nose, red eyes, sneezing and coughing, nose-blowing. He had a kit with various cold remedies, boxes of Kleenex and a small container which held several vials of an injectable medication. "Doc just give me a shot. I can't sing without it."

Well, here was my dilemma. This man obviously had a viral respiratory infection, and this compromised his ability to sing, but he also seemed very tense and anxious, and having worked often in the theatre with performers suffering from stage fright, I felt there seemed to be an element of this here. This was surprising in a performer of this caliber, but the combination of the cold and the pressure of another one-night performance certainly affected his usual bravado. Now, this man was a very decent person, appreciative of the fact that I had taken the time to come to see him. He explained that when his voice problem had occurred in the past his doctor had administered this medication ("An injection in the butt.") with very satisfactory results. I looked at the vials, there were three present, one missing, likely used previously. They were labeled "glyceryl guiacolate". Now, this is a well-known oral medication, it is contained in many over-the-counter cough mixtures. I had never, ever heard of this as an injectable compound. My immediate concern was this: what possible benefit would this have on a viral upper respiratory infection? I really felt unable to administer this as an injection, having no knowledge of this method of administration. Asking him about previous use, he stated his "doc" just gave him the shot and it worked fine.

At this point, the promoter poked his head through the door and demanded action. Pressure, but I was still not ready to comply. At that point, I undertook to call his own doctor, who had originally prescribed this stuff, a trick I had learned when treating people from out of town, often performers or hotel guests. I handed him the phone. "Get me your doc right now," I requested. He was, surprisingly, able to do this within almost five minutes. On the phone, his "doc" came through in a loud, clear southern accent. When I explained my problem with this unusual approach to his symptoms, the reply came back in a gruff drawl, but also in a kindly manner: "Just give him the shot in the ass, he'll sing like a bird!" He also explained, somewhat to my satisfaction, that his name was on the prescription box, that he had used this with effect in the past and, sensing my discomfort with the procedure, stated he would be responsible and I was not to worry, this said in a more professional tone.

Well, I gave him the "shot in the butt" (to the nurse's regret). I also asked him to breathe some steam (as there was an electric kettle handy), gargle with warm saline and add the nasal spray. I told him I was not familiar with such powerful medication and that these simple procedures would augment the effect. I told the support staff to brew him a strong cup of tea, stating this would help clear his bronchial tubes. I left him, mentioning how impressed I was with his doctor who knew him better than anyone else. I wished him well, and told him his "doc" was right: "once you get on stage you will sing like a bird!" And he did.

I was given a seat with a good view of the stage. The warm-up band who gave a very good, if slightly prolonged, performance gave way to the big man, the crowd now making a lot of noise! Any slight huskiness in his voice only added to the quality of his truly amazing performance. The flow of the hormones, adrenalin and cortisol, plus the placebo effect of the shot, saved the day!

Often, in the stress of the moment, ethical medical behavior can present a problem. The question of whether or not to administer a medication with which one has no information or experience, or simply to refuse to go along with the request, presented for me a bit of a crisis. Medical decisions can at times be a little like poker. Read the faces, listen to the comments, follow the gut reaction. As the song says: "You got to know when to hold 'em and when to fold 'em."

BAD MEMORIES

Many people will remember the dreadful polio epidemics of the thirties, forties and early fifties. I can recall, in 1937, that children were kept out of school until October twelfth, so my sister and I stayed at my grandmother's cottage to avoid contact with other children who might be infected. Indeed, my father (a general practitioner in Toronto), during the epidemic summer months, would often stay at the hospital if he had been in contact with an active case (which, unfortunately, occurred all too frequently), in fear he might carry the infection home to us. In that year, one of the most severe, there were 2544 cases, 109 deaths and 783 others who suffered residual paralysis. That in a city which was much less populous than today. This was a truly terrifying disease! In my early medical school years I was fortunate enough to become a member of a medical fraternity, several members of which had achieved high academic status, and one of the requirements was to report on medical research projects in our faculty. In my case, I had been informed that a Dr. Proctor at the school of hygiene was attempting to develop a medium which would support living tissue if kept at the appropriate temperature and supplied with oxygen. In his lab was a large blackboard, labelled at the top: "THE SOUP", with a long list of ingredients which were intended to supply adequate nourishment to sustain a living cell. This had had many modifications over the long, tedious process. At that time, the only way of growing viruses was in live animals, mostly rhesus monkeys imported from India, an expensive and frustrating procedure mostly sustained by The March of Dimes, a charity to support polio research. Over several visits, I was introduced to the progress being made to achieve the ability to culture living cells "in vitro", i.e., outside of a living animal. The attempts to develop a culture medium, which was intensively studied in a number of research centers was finally successfully achieved, allowing living cells to survive in a controlled medium. Cells from various human and animal sources were cultured so viral infections could be induced and studied. However, normal cell lines had limited growth potential, in that after several generations the cells died off, limiting the ability to achieve adequate cell mass to produce vaccines. At Johns Hopkins Hospital in 1951, a biopsy was obtained from a patient in their care. These were tumor cells, which, when introduced to the culture medium, thrived and grew in massive numbers. They were apparently not inhibited, as was the case with the many attempts to grow other cell lines. These human cancer cells, code named "He La", after the patient source, were widely distributed to any researcher who requested them. Because of their remarkable ability to reproduce, apparently in an immortal manner, they have achieved worldwide notoriety in medical research. They enabled the production of several important vaccines, and continue to be used widely in cancer and genetic investigations internationally.

In the mid-fifties, the polio virus could finally be grown in significant amounts using this cell line, which would allow researchers–like the well-known Dr. Jonas Salk–to extract enough viral material to formulate a vaccine from an inactivated (killed) virus, which when injected gave rise to an immune response in those vaccinated, protecting them from the disease.

In the summer of 1954, I was an intern at The Hospital for Sick Children in Toronto. Polio in its epidemic form was still very active, indeed, three of my close friends (all members of the swimming team at U of T), were stricken with bulbar polio, which attacks the upper part of the spinal cord, paralyzing the respiratory muscles, and without the ability to breathe recovery was almost non-existent. All these men were in perfect health; outstanding athletes. All had acquired their infections in widely-differing areas during summer employment, giving emphasis to the sporadic nature of this disease. All three died!

My duties were assigned to the infectious disease section, seventh floor. Dr. Crawford Anglin was our supervisor, at that time it was quite early in his career. Later, he became one of the outstanding pediatric infectious disease department heads at the hospital. It was summer and, of course, polio season. Although almost all of our admissions were gastroenteritis, which, frighteningly enough, could signal onset of polio, we had two memorable cases during my time there. Two thirteen-year-old girls were admitted, both had been swimming in the same pool in North Toronto. Both had fever and gastrointestinal symptoms, but had started to have problems speaking and, soon, breathing. They were admitted within three days of each other. Rapidly, their ability to breathe diminished and they became desperately ill, requiring respiratory assistance. In those days, the method employed was the Emerson respirator–the iron lung: a large metal cylinder which contained the patient, with only their head projecting from this frightening apparatus. As the pressure in the machine rose and fell breathing could be sustained, but with great difficulty. If the breathing was too fast or too slow, the acidity/alkalinity of the blood was altered. In those days, the measuring of blood gasses was slow and less accurate, while today these tests are done in minutes with any patient in respiratory distress. The first girl died within three days, as her disease worsened quickly. The other was able to be kept alive with tremendous effort by hospital staff. This was to me–a new, inexperienced doctor–a devastating experience I can still relive in my mind after all these years. At that time, the problem of cross-infection was of great concern (although it was later discerned that infection was transmitted via the gastro-intestinal system), any personal contact was considered dangerous. The result of this possibility of carrying the virus home was total isolation, even family! The young woman had several siblings and the danger that a visiting family member might acquire or transmit the disease had to be considered. The family was, therefore, not allowed to visit! My most poignant memories were of this child's mother standing on Elm Street across from the hospital, looking up at the window of the hospital room on the seventh floor, where her daughter could see her via a large round mirror above her head as she was forced to lie on her back in the machine, now almost completely paralyzed! That desperate woman stood there for hours, knowing her daughter could see her, while the mother could only wave.

Days later, she was unable to be sustained, and as with the other child, was overcome by this dreadful disease.

It is now taken for granted that polio can be eradicated (despite terrible opposition in some troubled countries), and both Salk and Sabin vaccines are now readily available. Several years later, when I had started my practice in family medicine, a young mother expressed strong opposition to my offer to administer the polio vaccine, holding the belief that it was not natural and possibly harmful! Although she seemed relatively well-educated and not unable to understand the benefits, she remained adamant. Well, at that point, I lost it. That a woman would not consider the wisdom of what was then modern medicine really hit me. How in the world could I possibly convince her that she was ill-informed? At first, I was almost ready to dismiss her from my practice, but to what end, and could I even do it? I asked her to return and bring her husband, as I had some information about the vaccine. She reluctantly complied and several days later showed up with child and husband. He was a quiet, somewhat recessive man with little to say, the wife doing most of the talking. It would take time, but I was bound and determined that this child would get the vaccine. I embarked on the history of the polio epidemics of the past and was not surprised that they came from a small town, as this disease is usually urban, and found in more densely populated areas. I told of the struggles to conquer this disease, finally resulting in a safe, effective method of prevention. I told her of my exposure to polio: losing friends and patients, as well as my family concerns (mostly my father's approach). Finally, I asked her how she would feel if she was the mother of the child who died of bulbar polio, standing alone on the street? She had sited religious beliefs in opposition, so I finalized by stating: "God helps those who help themselves." Long period of silence, then: "We'll do it." It was the husband speaking! This took a lot of time and fervor on my part, but I WON!

SHOW BIZ

In the fall of 1960, the O'Keefe Centre for the Performing Arts was opened in Toronto with much fanfare, as the initial production, Camelot, was to be the first presentation. This was a pre-Broadway endeavor, having been written by Fritz Loewe (music) and Alan Jay Lerner (book and lyrics). It was directed by the legendary Moss Hart. The cast included Richard Burton, Julie Andrews, Roddy McDowall and our own Canadian, Robert Goulet, in what became his first Broadway role. After the spectacular success of My Fair Lady, this writing team had the very best credentials. This was a big deal for the Toronto theatre world.

At that time, I was one of the physicians associated with the Royal York CPR Hotel, albeit a junior member, as my father, a long time Toronto Physician, and another senior doctor performed the occupational health program for employees and would from time to time be required to see guests who might require a physician. As might be expected, a number of these calls would come after-hours. Guess who would frequently be dispatched? I was not always pleased at the time, but it made for some very interesting encounters. It also happened that the theatre manager, one Bruce Corder (who brought extensive experience from the London theatre district), was a new neighbor and also a patient of mine. Although there was a CEO who oversaw the whole operation, Bruce was the hands-on manager who was there at all hours, dealing with the myriad problems of a large, new and untested facility.

Many older Torontonians recall the problems with this new production, faced as it was with the possibility of failure, and this was often reported in the press, which took delight in continuous criticism (although trying in some way to be supportive). Needless to say, the lights burned very late at the executive suite at the old Royal York! My call came about 2:00 a.m.; in those days there was no 911 call, you had to just get the doctor ASAP. This occurred several nights after the opening. The opening night performance ran to four and a half hours, with the expected run to be two hours and forty minutes! As I arrived, the scene was chaotic. Mr. Lerner was lying on the bed moaning, acutely ill. Mr. Hart took me to the toilet, which had just been filled with bright red blood!

An ambulance was summoned, transporting him at once, where he was treated in hospital for a severe bleeding duodenal ulcer. In the few intervening minutes awaiting transfer, I determined his hemoglobin (red blood count) was dangerously low. Off he went to the hospital with two members of the group who were close to him, and who had notified his family.

The stresses these performers endured were incredibly severe. At that point I had believed that show business was all excitement and success, with, of course, the occasional heartbreak. Now they were charged with cutting out almost two hours of material, meanwhile, the show was running. Also, the demands on the performers, all of whom were seasoned, experienced and extremely capable, were enormous. Imagine having learned all your lines; rehearsed the dialogue, music and choreography; just to have it changed abruptly, almost on a nightly basis! Remember Jiminy Cricket in the Disney film Pinocchio? "Hey Diddely-dee, an actor's life for me?" I don't think so! I had never before realized the incredibly hard work and dedication demonstrated by these extraordinary people. Alan Lerner, who was an absolute master of lyrics (and who, incidentally, was a former Harvard classmate of President John F. Kennedy), had been through a difficult divorce, and the stresses inflicted by that were compounded many times by the responsibility of making this show a success. All of the principals in the production were present during this crisis, and the fact that Mr. Lerner was still barking instructions as he was wheeled out to the hospital spoke to the motivation to succeed in this remarkable group. When I left they had mostly returned to the job at hand, having reassured him that they would complete the day's proposed changes, perhaps not fully aware of the severe nature of this illness.

The seriousness of the situation was complicated by another problem. As Lerner was recovering and taking more responsibility in affecting the ongoing changes, I got a call to see Moss Hart to discuss a new concern. He had avoided mentioning the onset of episodic headaches as: "there were enough problems already." However, these headaches were now interfering with his heavy work-load. Now, the dilemma. His headaches were moderate-to-severe, located in the upper occipital region, midline, almost at the crown, and associated with this he would feel rather marked fatigue. However, he would recover from these episodes and carry on with work. As is well known from his book "Act One," he had previous stress-related episodes of anxiety and depression, his whole life had been in theatre, where he had honed his tremendous talent in writing, directing and acting. Such afflictions are fairly common in the extremely gifted in the upper echelons of the theatre community. However, Mr. Hart, although tired, stressed and at times quite angry with some of the circumstances affecting this endeavor (i.e., the attitude of the Toronto press), as well as the technical glitches common in any theatre–especially one so new–had kept intensely focused on the work at hand; his abilities in reshaping a theatrical production such as this was legendary. He had simply ignored the symptoms. His past history was vague, but he had been warned of a heart condition. Now, here was the enigma: although the pain he had described was in no way typical of angina (heart pain due to insufficient blood flow to the heart muscle), it definitely was not psychosomatic. I needed help. I contacted Dr. Alf Kerwin, chief of cardiology at my teaching hospital. It was helpful that Dr. Kerwin was a theatre buff and had read Moss Hart's book. Sensing my concern, he responded at once. The result of this consultation was that there was evidence found of some myocardial damage; a heart attack had occurred and he had worked through it! He was hospitalized and treated by Dr. Kerwin, who brought my attention to the fact that heart pain can be very deceiving, a lesson I never forgot and which influenced my assessment of this frequent complaint all my medical life. It was very helpful that Dr. Kerwin was an aficionado of both London's West End and the New York theatre scene, and had read and enjoyed Moss Hart's "Act One", as mentioned above. As a result, he had gained his patient's respect and attention towards following reasonable treatment plans. Remember, in those days there were not the invasive cardiac treatments we enjoy today, no bypass procedures (open heart surgery) or stents modifying blood flow to the heart. This demonstrates the importance of doctor-patient relationships, in that the consultant fully comprehended the nature of the demands on the director, and indeed had seen one of the amended performances. Thus, the patient, now aware that the doctor fully appreciated his responsibilities as a director, was able to comply with and adjust to the medical restrictions to the activities permitted. The result was a fairly good recovery, and the ability to carry the production of "Camelot" to its ultimate Broadway success.

One of the other less-severe problems that arose throughout the Toronto experience was Julie Andrews' shoulder pain. In each performance, she was required to vigorously wave a large flag on a heavy ornate flagstaff. Wincing with pain at each wave while continuing the herculean task of relearning new lyrics and dialogue almost nightly, she needed a solution. The Royal York doctors had diagnosed tendonitis, and arranged treatment which including physiotherapy, but the greatest help came from the production team, props and costumes. They redesigned a very lightweight staff and smaller flag, so the shoulder was spared. This was quickly facilitated by the ever-present manager, Bruce Corder.

The wild ride of the grand opening of the O'Keefe (later Hummingbird, and now Sony Centre), will be remembered by all involved in the events. But to be a fly on the wall during some pretty dramatic events, and to be included in the process was an extraordinary experience. I was deeply impressed and proud of all the medical personnel, particularly the staff at the hospital who so competently and quickly provided excellent care. The expressed gratitude of the family members was touching, notably Moss Hart's wife Kitty Carlisle–a legend herself– who flew up immediately at the news of her husband's illness and quietly and sincerely thanked us for our efforts. What a privilege to interact with these amazing people away from the glare of the Marquee.

SEX-ED FOR THE COMMUNITY

In the immediate years after finishing my residency training new patients were slow in coming, even though I had association with my father's practice. Recall that in those days, prenatal and well-baby care was about the only proactive medical management protocol used in practice, as patients usually only came to the doctor if they were ill or injured. However, I–as did other physicians associated with our teaching hospital–worked in the Out-Patients Department. We would attend clinic on one or two mornings from 8:00 to 12:00, where we were expected to provide care for those unable to afford a private practitioner. In fact, in the earliest days, I could even spend up to three mornings offering service. These were teaching experiences for senior medical students and rotating interns. Our job as graduated, practicing doctors was to teach and supervise these young men and women. For our contribution to the hospital, we were afforded admitting privileges and the use of the Emergency Department to do simple procedures and deliver urgent care, such as acute illnesses, suturing, and other injuries including the management of simple fractures. Also, when they were short of staff I would work in the obstetrical clinic, as I was interested in delivering babies, having moonlighted during my second residency year delivering babies for physicians who wanted a night or weekend off. If the senior teaching staff were satisfied with your performance, they would direct more work your way, thus, an eager young MD could gain valuable experience. Our work was always monitored by the department heads who were available for consultation. My friend Peter was also a brand-new starting family doctor in Toronto's West End, where a number of more senior physicians were already well-established associates of our Toronto Western Hospital. Between the two of us, we got to do a number of extra obstetrical cases.

Remember, in those days, a constant problem was unwanted or illegitimate pregnancies. There was no birth control, the pill had not arrived, condoms were usually of poor quality and a teen could not easily obtain them. The diaphragm was a poor substitute, requiring a visit to the doctor. So, when an unfortunate teenager got pregnant or a marriage had not occurred, there was trouble!

The sexual information available to children and, most importantly, late-teens was almost nonexistent, and what was available was fraught with misinformation and judgmental attitudes, to the point of bigotry. Indeed, in some cases, a pregnant teen could become an outcast, even occasionally being forced to leave the family home! On more than one occasion, a father has told his daughter to leave the house, having brought disgrace to the family. When pressed for how much information the child had received re avoiding pregnancy, often the response was that she had been told it was all her responsibility!

Well, during the first two years of our practices Peter and I probably managed more illegitimate children than regular patient deliveries. The reason was that we were both known to the more senior staff, who frequently referred these young women to us as they knew we would accept them as patients.

About this time, my Toronto Western associate and I both had our own young children, and babysitting was hard to come by. I had an in with the Hospital for Sick Children's nursing school, where one could often get a reliable sitter, but not always. Peter's wife was a nurse, so at times they really needed a sitter when they both were busy. I happened to have a really nice seventeen-year-old as a patient who had been evicted by her dad and was staying with an older sister, but the older sister had a new baby herself and my patient was sleeping on the couch. I knew my friend had a rather large west-end house, not yet full of kids. I suggested they offer a room to my patient, who would try to continue school but who could babysit several evenings a week so his wife could do her evening shifts. Room and board and spending money, but most of all a sympathetic, understanding family. This arrangement worked very well for all. I remained the doctor, providing prenatal care, then delivery and immediate after-care. In those days, the ability of a young mother to keep her baby was almost never considered, so the usual answer was adoption. Keep in mind that at that time abortion was totally illegal.

The Children's Aid and the involvement of a very kind young woman lawyer were, for Peter and me, invaluable in helping with adoption proceedings. My wife and I had an opportunity to have another young woman come and stay in our third-floor extra bedroom. My friend managed her obstetrical care, and we had acquired the extra help needed. This one particular teen was a true find! She had been sent to stay with a rather strict aunt in a small town, a situation she hated, as she was truly treated almost as if she were a servant. There were no others in town with whom she could associate; she was lonely and miserable. Also, she would have to change schools. When she heard of our offer she was very pleased. She had younger brothers, whom she missed. We had three sons and lived on a street with lots of kids, so when she arrived she just fit in so very well. She was quite a good athlete, not a beauty but a really nice-looking seventeen-year-old. She quickly bonded with the boys and almost reached term before she stopped being involved in active sports. Indeed, she became a temporary "big sister" and really was considered one of the family. It was a regular occurrence in our house that the neighborhood kids would congregate in our kitchen, munch on endless cookies and talk. It was a revelation to them that this young woman had become pregnant without planning to do so. It was also very apparent that this experience was hard for her, and that she was not a bad person. This kid was amazing, in that she had no hesitation in explaining that she did not really know anything about avoiding pregnancy. Yes, she had had sex, but it had all happened so fast that she hardly realized what had truly occurred, and that it "wasn't that great". Wide-eyed wonder from the younger ones at this first-hand information, and when the initial giggling and silly talk abated more and more relevant questions arose. What would happen to the baby? How would she feel? A kid on the block had an adopted sibling: more discussion. There were some complaints, but when, at a local cocktail party, a parent questioned the wisdom of what we had done, my wife and I explained that it was overall a very enlightening experience for the children, and the objections faded. We did, however, have one rather difficult situation arise. A boy from several blocks away happened to be on our front lawn. He had not been aware of our "big sister" and made some very disparaging remarks about her getting "knocked up"; very embarrassing for her and for the several immediate neighbor kids present. I was upstairs, it was summer and all the windows were open. I heard raising of voices: "You can't say that!" More epithets, then… "SMACK", followed by screaming and crying. The boy who had made the remarks was running home. It wasn't long before he returned with his mother, who was demanding that my son (the oldest), the one who had whopped this guy, be punished for his actions. As I was coming out the front door, this woman was beset by almost all of those young people present loudly repeating what this boy had said. Our stoic babysitter stood silently by, now almost at term, obviously embarrassed. Having learned what remarks had been made and that they were totally unacceptable, I suggested she take him home, as he would not be welcome here. She, rather sheepishly, left. The kids all gathered around our "big sister" and gave her a big hug.

She was the third of the unwed moms who stayed with us over the early years. For many years after she left for home she wrote to us at Christmas with cards and occasional letters, to return in a way to a family very much affected by the whole experience. She graduated from university, and later married and had two children. All the local kids, now mostly grown, still talk of the times spent around the kitchen table. For years, they knew they could get accurate information, not just on sexual questions, but on many other medical topics. There is nothing like first-hand experience, open and honest sources of knowledge, and having their questions answered. To think, we are still conflicted about good quality reproductive teaching many years later.

A REALLY BAD CASE OF MEASLES

While cycling or driving through Central Toronto, I am often reminded of past experiences that remain etched in my memory. Recently, cycling up Parliament Street, I passed an older building in Moss Park which sparked a recall. As I continue to follow health issues, the recently discussed "Determinants of Health"(often referred to when managing health care policy), points to poverty and mental illness as major factors. This prompted the following story:

A very cold late January evening, only one year into starting my practice, I received an urgent call to see a very sick baby. The call had come from a woman whom I had attended in clinic, who noted that her neighbor in the next apartment had a constantly-crying baby who was also coughing violently. She had asked if she could help, but the mother declined stating: "it was just a bad cold".

The neighbor then noted the child had become quiet, prompting her to ask again if she could help. At this point, the mother seemed more concerned, as the child had suddenly become more ill, now only coughing with difficulty, and this was associated with marked congestion and labored breathing. Hence, the call to me, as my number was available.

She was in a third-floor walkup in a still-standing red brick building (although evidently scheduled for demolition, as had already occurred in the adjacent structures). I entered, noting the entrance door was held open by a door-stop. Aware of the apartment number, I started up the stairs. This place had not been well kept, and was also extremely over-heated, so as I had hurriedly reached the upper floor I was drenched in sweat. This state of warmth was a result of not only coming from a warm house in a warm car, but the fact that I was wearing a brand-new winter coat, of which I was very proud. It was sheepskin, quite heavy, and worn over a tweed jacket!

As I entered the apartment, I realized that it was perhaps even hotter than the corridor. I was shocked by the situation. In front of a small TV, a large unkempt man in an undershirt sat with a beer in his hand. He did not look up or in any way acknowledge my arrival although I was only a few feet away. The mother, who seemed distraught and also smelled of alcohol, accepted my presence and indicated that the baby was in a small, dark bedroom. Now, where to put my coat? There was absolutely no place that I would consider leaving it as the man was on the couch, the dining table was covered with dirty dishes, one small chair had stuff draped on it and the coffee table was covered with empty beer bottles! I entered the bedroom; more heat. On a small cot was a brown cotton padded quilt, the kind used to protect furniture when moving, or which might be hung in the elevator as protection. A small, beet-red head projected from this covering, which I immediately removed, revealing a very young child almost too hot to touch, a red macular rash over his upper body and very severe respiratory congestion, still trying to cough! He wore a diaper, only slightly damp, and when I took his temperature it was 105.4! This kid had a very severe case of red measles. I could not get a satisfactory history of immunization, and the mother seemed not to understand the potential seriousness of this situation. At this point, the neighbor appeared, checking that I had arrived. We conferred and she, being a fairly sensible woman, agreed that the child was in need of hospital care. She vouched for the fact that these parents were in fact common-law, and she expressed doubt that he was the true father as he had just taken up with her in recent months. Pretty obvious that this pair would not be competent in managing this very sick child.

Having instructed the mother to gently cool the child by wiping him down with a damp cloth, I examined the baby. Subsequently, I went to the bathroom to wash my hands. No soap, no towels, but worst of all was the powerful ammonia stench of dirty diapers, which were several inches deep in the bathtub! Boy, was I eager to get out of there. I was almost relieved that the phone was out of service, so I was able to go next door to phone for an ambulance, but not before finally removing my coat! I instructed the hospital that a severe case of red measles was on its way.

Fortunately, the ambulance did arrive quite quickly and the attendants, who were also shocked at the deplorable conditions, dressed the child in a clean, small gown, continuing to attempt to lower the fever. Off they went, providing what oral fluids they could.

When I arrived home (having mostly driven with the windows open), I changed my clothes and washed thoroughly, then called the hospital. I did this as I had not been able to write an admission note to the ER physician. By the time I had finally arrived home, the patient had been in ER for slightly more than one hour, and due to the cold winter temperature and the attendants care, the fever was much less severe, and with rehydration there was some improvement. Now came the shock. Finally, the charge nurse agreed to let me speak to the resident on call. He rather callously stated that when they had finished with the work-up, they would be sending the patient home! I tried to explain that the home situation was totally unable to cope with managing this child. "Sorry, but that's your problem," was the curt reply. Now what? Fortunately, I remembered that my very close friend was in his final year as chief resident in cardiology. I called him via "locating", getting him when he was finally free. After recounting this story of the total dysfunction in the child's home, he was annoyed at the cavalier way I was treated: as another GP dumping a patient into the hospital. He was incredibly helpful, as his position and ability were well known to all, especially in the ER where he spent considerable time. Soon all was sorted out, I had expressed concern re possible complications of red measles (i.e., brain involvement), and the desperate need for social services, if not the Children's Aid, in dealing with the child's environment. My friend stepped in immediately and called social services, spoke to the medical chief resident, and chewed out the intern who was rather unhelpful when I tried to explain the circumstances. The child was admitted to the infectious disease unit where I had worked as an intern three years before, so I was made welcome to call and follow the outcome. Fortunately, Miss Palmer, the legendary head nurse who had helped us interns through the terrible polio epidemic of the summer of 1954 (when we lost two young girls to bulbar polio), remembered me. After I again explained the circumstances, it was she who made sure that the social services followed this child, who was eventually placed with the Children's Aid, and the mother was referred to the psychiatric service at The Toronto General Hospital.

It was with great relief that I, as an inexperienced new family doctor, could draw upon friends and associates to help solve a complex problem.

NORMAL MORE COMMON THAN ABNORMAL

In the fifties and early sixties in Toronto, almost all babies were delivered in hospitals. Our training in obstetrics did not include home delivery. While we were aware that home deliveries were common in the UK and Europe, and certainly were the rule in third-world countries, it was not the practice here.

One of my very memorable patients was a woman in her mid-twenties, with whom I had a number of polemic encounters. A bright, articulate employee in a publishing company, a third generation African-Canadian and a University of Toronto graduate in English and History, she first presented with a minor ankle injury due to running. As she had insurance (no OHIP at that time), she insisted on an X-ray. It took some convincing that this was not really necessary, as it was only a minor sprain. I finally prevailed, by pointing out that somebody's money was being wasted. Similar encounters had occurred, one with respect to a bad cold, which did not need penicillin. This patient was a tall, imposing woman, well dressed and attractive. She never, from our first meeting on, addressed me by anything other than my first name: David. In those days, the use of the term "doctor" was the norm. She was in no way disrespectful, and as she was only a few years my junior, I was comfortable with this. She possessed a great sense of humor, and I recall one of her stories.

After graduation, she had traveled to Europe, and following this to Africa, where she spent some time in Nigeria teaching English and volunteering at a local hospital. Laughing, she stated: "Do you know how weird it was for me there? My accent was different, in many instances my beliefs were different, but I looked the same as everybody else! Big change from here, but I'm glad to be home." I have often thought about that statement, as there were fewer people of color in the city in those times. We did not seem to think of racist differences as much then, but she reminded me that there will always be racism in some form or other, and she felt it was her responsibility to accept it and rise above it. Her humorous approach to this was: "In a thousand years, if humanity survives, black;

white; red; yellow will all be so mixed, everybody will be a neutral mud colour, so it won't make any difference."

Not long after this visit, she presented with the statement that she might be pregnant. Period overdue, feeling tired and slightly nauseated at times, it was established that she was expecting. Before I could propose an outline of management, she gave me her very definite plan.

I was aware she was not married, but she, sensing my sensitivity concerning this, immediately reassured me that she had an outstanding partner, and she was delighted with the prospect of motherhood. In those days this was somewhat unusual, but I was prepared to have her present her proposal. Well, she started out with: "I will be having the baby at home! I will keep working and now, of course, be getting married." Her partner, a teacher (who, by the way, was white), was also delighted at the news. Well! My attempts to convince her that home deliveries were almost non-existent in those days fell on deaf ears. It took a very long time to explain that there were no available protocols or facilities for home care as, at that time, the only arrangements would be an ambulance ride to the nearest hospital if the baby was coming precipitously. I finally had to tell her I simply would not attempt this under any circumstances. I explained that all the facilities to manage obstetrical emergencies were available in the hospital, so any risk to baby or mother would be kept at a minimum. My mind raced over all the what-ifs that occupy the mind of those who are about to attend a birth; that is, the management of the many possible abnormal, sometimes even disastrous, outcomes. She was upset by the likelihood of any interference with a "perfectly natural process," which to her would be unacceptable.

When I brought out my standard prenatal protocol sheets, her observation was that it was a total waste of paperwork. She objected to routine blood and urine testing, weights and blood pressure charting. "Why don't I just call you when I think the baby is coming, I'll go to the hospital and get this over with." Now, I must say, although this was confrontational and did require extra time in long explanations, she did maintain a certain element of humor, such that I found it hard to even be annoyed. We carried on with this give-and-take all through the pregnancy. Of course, she continuously admonished me because I never elicited one finding that was not entirely normal.

Her last office visit was three days after her due date. Impatiently, she asked: "When is this going to be over?" In those days, before the luxury of ultrasound imaging, estimating the date of delivery was pretty inaccurate. She was still at work and as she was, as noted, a tall, lean, athletic woman, she did look to be less at term than most would at this stage. I gave her all the instructions re informing me of the warning signs of onset of labor. The baby had not yet dropped, so I felt there might be more time before delivery, which did not please her. Four days later, while I was in the office, a call came that she had gone to the hospital. I called back almost at once, but got no answer. I called the hospital, the case room nurse said she had arrived some time earlier and that I had better get there soon! Making quick arrangements with the patients in the waiting room (fortunately all were women and fully compliant with my rather hasty departure, all seemed somewhat excited about the impending delivery), I left. Late afternoon traffic! Slow trip to hospital. Annoyed that she did not inform me sooner. It seemed every little thing impeded my progress: parking delay, slow elevator… Damn. As I got off the elevator whom do I see sitting in a gurney in the hall outside the delivery room but my patient! Beside her, chatting amiably, the head nurse, who had actually delivered the baby. A colleague who had just finished his case had checked her, and also the baby who was in the bassinette crying lustily. All was in perfect order. She had a full-term, normal delivery, with no problems or complications. Whew!

With relief I approached, wondering just what to say, she, with a huge smile and actually laughing, said: "See, if only you had done what I wanted in the first place, we could have avoided all this nonsense!" Her husband-to-be turned out to be a terrific guy, a high school teacher and football coach, who, incidentally, was in agreement with my plan all along. This remarkable couple had been busy. She, because there was no maternity leave in those days, had quit her job and already applied for a teaching position in a school near where her prospective husband was employed. My next encounter was with her mother, also a tall, imposing woman, who looked more like an older sister than her mother. "She's quite a handful," she remarked to me. "You must have had the patience of Job."

A TALE OF TWO POLICEMEN

In the early days of my obstetrical practice, prospective fathers were usually excluded from the delivery room. It seemed to me a rather Victorian concept, but that was the accepted protocol. During my wife's first thirty-two-hour prolonged labor (resulting in a c-section), I was sent home three times! I accepted this at the time, but over the ensuing years the concept was modified by a number of younger physicians, and the rule was relaxed.

In my early practice, I was delivering two to three babies per month and tended to spend extra time in the case room, eager to gain experience in the management of obstetrical emergencies. Although these events are rare, they do occur. I did have to face two catastrophic births. One, a severe hydrocephalic (brain deformity) which resulted in the loss of the baby, and a still-birth due to a cord abnormality which occurred before the mother could get to the hospital. On a rare occasion, a skilled, highly-trained obstetrician was able to avert a seriously bad outcome in a patient, possibly saving her life. It was a comforting fact that in a large teaching hospital help was always at hand. I admired the colleagues who practiced in remote areas with little or no immediate support. Hence, I had some concern about having a father in the room, which resulted in three patients instead of two.

On one rather memorable occasion, a nurse and I were standing at the nurse's station when we noticed a large man standing beside his wife on a gurney just outside the delivery room, he was putting handcuffs on his and her wrists. This was not my patient. "Oh-oh, trouble," says the nurse! Down the hall came the attending obstetrician, a very serious, conservative man, who had refused the husband, an impressive plain-clothed policeman, attendance in the delivery room. The nurses had warned the husband about the intransigence of this senior physician, but he was determined to accompany her, hence the handcuffs. The doctor, a professor in the medical faculty whom we all admired for his unflappable nature and skill in managing acute obstetrical emergencies, spoke quietly: "I hope you have good luck in the delivery. I usually require two hands to do a good job, one hand may not be enough." He then started to walk away down the hall. At this point the next contraction came, signaling rather definite progress toward actual delivery. Well, the wife let out a shriek and yanked very hard on the handcuffs. "Get these G.D. things off!" The big cop unlocked the cuffs and sheepishly went to the waiting room. I found out later he was presented with a healthy baby boy; well worth the wait!

Shortly after this experience I was visited by a young woman in my practice who was expecting. She was the wife of a young police officer, a very nice man excited to be expecting their first baby. As we went through the full prenatal workup he was always present and very compliant and supportive. At about midterm he very respectfully and with some reservation requested he be permitted to attend the delivery. With the memory of the experience of the other police officer, and the fact that the exclusion of fathers was being reconsidered by a number of my younger colleagues, I decided to comply. The labor started as expected, I explained that the first baby was usually a little slower than subsequent deliveries. At the hospital, he stayed with her the whole time being very supportive and empathetic. When ready for the delivery room, both were quite tired, as expected, and just prior to delivery an epidural anesthetic was decided upon as the pain was severe. The husband had been sent to get a cap, mask, gown and shoe covers. He had come from work and had worn his uniform, having stashed all his police paraphernalia in a locker, including his gun, etc. He had a problem getting the turquoise paper shoe covers over his big black boots. Because the anesthetist was monitoring the patient on her right side, and the case room nurse was standing on her left, the father was positioned immediately behind me in a fairly tight corner between the window and a projection from the wall. With the epidural relieving the discomfort, the baby started to come quickly. I was busy delivering the head with the usual gush of amniotic fluid, blood and a small lateral tear. Out came the baby! I had just placed the baby, with the cord attached, on mom's abdomen, when I looked down. Below the delivery table is a large basin with sterile towels. The mom's feet and legs were covered by green drapes which partly obscured my view of the father. Suddenly, I saw the basin start to move slowly to my right. And pushing it were two large, turquoise paper-covered boots! I suddenly realized dad had quietly fainted and was sliding down feet-first, and when his bottom hit the floor his head toppled forward toward the basin, which had been partly pushed aside. I was just able to get my left foot under his chin to avert his head hitting the floor and/or the basin. He rolled over, and the anesthetist was able to drag him off to the side, and as he was only unconscious for a very brief period, revive him in time to recover and see the baby. I was able to deliver the placenta and repair the small tear, meanwhile, mom was so excited to get the baby she had no idea what had gone on in the corner. The anesthetist, a cool guy with a great sense of humor, got dad up to see the outcome! All good. We left it up to the dad to tell his wife what happened. It surprised me at the time that a big, healthy policeman would faint. I had certainly not expected this, but I found out later he had come off a long shift and was very tired (as was the mom), dehydrated and emotionally exhausted, so I should have anticipated a problem. Lesson learned.

In the future, I was very careful to prepare the prospective father or other observer, and not have them behind me, I would put them in a position to be very close to the mother. The new birthing process is so different now; the procedure, the ambiance, all changed. And all for the good!

UNIVERSITY ADDRESS

Address given to the University of Toronto Graduating Class in Medicine 2014 by Dr. David Smith, President of the Class of 1954

Sixty years ago I spoke on behalf of the great Class of 5T4, and I wish to express my appreciation to past and present members for trusting me to do so. Ten years ago I commented on the Health care system. What does one do when embedded in a large, complex, bureaucratic, politicized organization? Keep working on it! Dr. Danielle Martin now a well known Toronto Family Doc has eloquently spoken out on this topic. Good luck to Dr. Bob Bell our new Deputy Minister of Health!

After sixty years primary care, and what a privilege this has been, some simple lessons I have learned. Three words come to mind: CARE, ASK, LISTEN.

Care from the word 'caritas' meaning care in the full sense of the word to include 'Attentiveness' and 'Respect'. You do not have to like your patient, but must understand how they got to their present state. And don't forget to be polite, your mother taught you that. And simple kindness, the basis of ongoing, palliative, supportive, and end of life care.

Very quickly the patient senses that a physician truly demonstrates these qualities! Think about it, these thing cost nothing! If every caregiver, doctor, nurse, receptionist, anyone involved in health care, behaved this way it would smooth over the myriad frustrating problems that plague us trying to get through a busy day. How often does one hear that a caregiver was rude or inattentive to a patient's needs? Poor communication skills often drive people to the 'Alternative Medicine' field, sometimes effective, often not, and occasionally harmful. A study at the Harvard Business School proposes that the most important skills in future will be social and emotional intelligence.

Next is 'ASK', open ended relevant questions, not the yes/no algorithms on the computer. And most important …'LISTEN'! Sir William Osler stated " If you listen, the patient will often give you the diagnosis".

Ask and listen are the basis for the management of most mental health issues which presently seem to be overwhelming the health care system, certainly in my field of primary care.

Finally the 'Elephant in the Room'. Were cannot function without our I-phone,I -pad and computer. Think Epocrates, Up to Date, Medline, Chochrane Collaboration and the proliferating 'EKR's'. I'm told that IBM's Watson can out diagnose most doctors! These are all amazing instruments of connectivity and information, BUT when you are one-on-one with a patient who has a problem, PLEASE address the person , not the machine!

BOTTOM LINE

[1] Key words CARE…ASK…LISTEN.
[2] Keep the 'Elephant' in perspective, address concerns about confidentiality, unwanted, harmful or useless information.
[3] The most important part of your 'remuneration' in life is the gratitude and appreciation of those for whom you have provided service, and the hope that somehow over the years, you may have made a difference.

EPILOGUE

"TO CURE SOMETIMES, TO TREAT
OFTEN, TO COMFORT ALWAYS."

Over the many years of patient contact, I have learned that establishing rapport with the patient is of prime importance. Communication in the fullest sense, that is the the ability to fully establish mutual trust, so that occult information is kept to a minimum. Observation, body language, talking, correct examination techniques, appropriate touching [hugs and hand holding], comprehending attitudes and beliefs, thus achieving an emotional connection that would be acceptable and comforting, greatly enhance the ability to provide effective care.

The words of Hippocrates say it all!

To my readers, family, associates, students, colleagues, patients and friends, thanks for listening…David.

ACKOWLEDGEMENTS

I wish to thank my wife Marlene,and cousin John Uren,for their strong encouragement and support. I also need to recognize my many friends and colleagues in The Department of Family and Community Medicine and those in Student Services, University of Toronto.

David R. F. Smith Bio

Dr. Smith graduated in medicine in 1954 from the University
of Toronto.

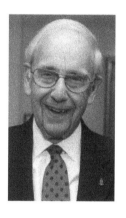

He completed residency
training at The Toronto Western
Hospital, now part of the the
University Health Network, and
the Sunnybrook Health Sciences
Centre, then DVA, Hospital,
entering Family Practice in 1956. He joined the staff
of The Toronto Western Hospital working in the Out
Patients Department. After ten years in private practice
in downtown Toronto in association with his father
Dr. Arthur Smith, a long time general practitioner, he was
asked to join a pilot group of primary care physicians, who
would form the first Family Practice teaching Unit, then
a new Department of the University of Toronto Faculty

of Medicine. It is of interest that at the present time this Department of Family and Community Medicine has become the largest Primary Care teaching Facility in the world, with approximately fifteen hundred members in the greater Toronto area and throughout Ontario. During the early teaching years he developed special interests in Student Medicine, Tropical and Parasitic Disease, and Palliative care. He received his Certification from the College of Family Physicians of Canada in 1971 and in 1985 became a Fellow of the College of Family Physicians of Canada. He was The Director of The University of Toronto Student Health Services from 1984 to 1996. He has been associated with the teaching faculty as associate professor in the Department. He is the permanent president of his graduating class of 1954. He retired after sixty years of active practice, in 2014. By writing of a few of his early experiences he softened the withdrawal from the demands of practice and the struggle to keep abreast of the myriad new developments in medicine.